askROCCO
Uncensored: Volume I

by
Rocco Castellano, CPFT
Syndicated Fitness Columnist

askROCCO Uncensored: Volume 1
An askROCCO Media Book

askROCCO Media™
8022 South Rainbow Blvd, Suite 219
Las Vegas, NV 89139

rocco@roccocastellano.com (email)
www.roccocastellano.com (www)

Photography for cover design by Gina Hartman
Cover design by Aspen Bessinger for askROCCO Media™.
aspen@1260productions.com

ISBN 13: 978-1494261634
ISBN 10: 1494261634

Comments from askROCCO readers

- *First I want to say I enjoy reading all of the info and suggestions you provide.*
  --Jo

- *Just wanted to voice my utter love for your article and intolerance for the fat and lazy. I couldn't agree with you more.*
  I once was a fat kid, but educated myself about diet and exercise (and actually abided by what I learned). I am now a svelte, sexy young lady (yes, even you bought me a drink a while back - thanks, btw).
  No one has to be fat. The fat love to make excuses for their laziness, when all it really comes down to is ignorance and gluttony. Thanks for putting it to 'em straight. Some call you rude, but "honest" would be a better description. Keep it comin'!
  --Amanda

- *I don't have a question - just wanted to give you a pat on the back about being a personal trainer and not a nutritionist. I am also a personal trainer and find that a lot of trainers do give nutritional advice that they should not be giving. I hear them talk all the time about diet and supplements and so often I just want to say something like "unless you have a degree in nutrition, I think should keep*

your mouth shut." So, I just wanted to commend you on that.
--Jen

* *I really get a kick out of your column with your straightforward approach to the obesity problem all around us. I work hard to stay in decent shape and I shouldn't let it bother me but it really does when I see an unbelievably obese person driving around in the store at Sam's and their eye's glaze over when they see them handing out food samples just so they can roll up to add to the problem.*
Can't even stand up to stuff their pie hole. Do you think that a lot of this obesity may be because of other issues (Mental/Emotional)? The other day as I sat eating my vegi-wrap and I noticed 7 out of every 10 women shopping were grossly obese. It's a shame especially when they say things like, "I'm OK with it what's your problem?"
Good luck with your article and please from all us guys who still enjoy looking at the nice shapely well-built women of America out there, keep telling it like it is.
--John

* *I just have to respond to this kid from India with "no time" to work out. Either you want it, or you don't. Besides working 50 hours a week at a bank, I also attend night school full time (4 classes per semester). Basically, I get off work and head to school, then get home about 9pm. Then what? The gym is what, about 3 to 4 nights a week and once on the weekend. I usually work out from 9:30 to 11 or so, then*

eat and hit the shower. Yeah I know it's bad to eat that late at night but I have no problems with weight gain in bad areas; I do enough cardio to combat that. I'm not single either, I have a wife and kid, and ride/race motorcycles on weekends. So, the problem is not enough time.... It's time management and the desire to be in shape. Some people are too lazy to get up off their asses and take a simple walk outside, but they complain of their love handles and shortness of breath. It's amazing, you can go just about anywhere and you'll be surrounded by 75% of people that are overweight. It's outrageous. More of them should start listening to you, and start taking action for their own sake.
--Phil

- *I think your column needs to be updated more frequently. I need 'Ask Rocco' more than once a week.*
  --Jessica

- *Rocco, I love your straightforward approach to exercise and nutrition. You clearly state that balancing your intake, reducing your calories, and daily exercise is the way to fitness. Thanks for being Rocco.*
  --Kelly

Chris Snider, editor of the Weekly Juice in Des Moines, Iowa, for taking the chance that Iowans might even get my sense of humor and creating the path for my column becoming syndicated. I need to thank my many readers in all my markets that keep me in business and keep me on my toes with some of the craziest questions I've ever been asked. Thanks for being out there.

People who have helped me get askROCCO Media off the ground and become a fitness information force. Thank you to Bill and Charlotte Vermillion for putting in countless hours in preparing the askROCCO Media™ Business Plan and placing my needs even before theirs on many occasions. Without them I may have given up; they are truly an inspiration and an intellectual force to be reckoned with. Stacy Reilly, although she doesn't know it, kept me going on the right path and has been the anvil on which I forged my askROCCO ideas; thank you.

Friends and Family:
Edward Bogosian for being there even when he couldn't, and always keeping me in his prayers. Christina Cavallo, for always being there. My brother Anthony, basically for being my brother. Thank you Melissa and Brian Pitchford, for allowing me to be the Official Personal Trainer for Miss Michigan USA™ and Miss Ohio USA™ and being my friends through thick and thin. We know there's been a lot of thick. Matthew Bryzcki, a great fitness author, who inspired me to get what I know down on paper and published my first chapter in a Publication called *Maximize your Training* ©1998 Contemporary Books.

There are so many other people I want to thank. You know who you are and I thank you.

To all my readers, my family and friends

CONTENTS

Acknowledgements

There would be no askROCCO if it weren't for some very important people. Without askROCCO there wouldn't be this book. I want to say a great big thank-you to Gary Burbank, the greatest comedic talent on radio. Thank you for allowing me to be a part of The Gary Burbank Show for eight and a half years giving me the opportunity to establish askROCCO as a brand. I'll never forget that fateful day playing Golf at Hickory Sticks and hearing you say, " I think we should have a segment called ASK ROCCO," and the rest is history.

There would not be an askROCCO brand as eminent as it is without the undying fortitude that Ran Mullins of Cleriti.com has demonstrated over the two years it took to create askROCCO. Everything that you see that is askROCCO I owe to Ran Mullins' creative brain. Ran's drive for perfection not only brought the askROCCO Media image to the masses, he created materials beyond our wildest dreams. He truly is an Artist/Entrepreneur and has proved that more times than I can count. Thank you. Please contact Ran at: http://www.cleriti.com/ran

Obviously, without the askROCCO column I wouldn't have the fan base that prompted me to create this publication. So hats off to Beryl Love, who is now Executive Editor of USA TODAY Network National News Desk but back when I was in Cincinnati was the editor in chief or cappo de editor tutti of CIN Weekly for having the vision and the balls for allowing my column to grace the pages of CiN Weekly. Forever I'll be thankful for his friendship, guidance and ability to take risks with an Italian boy from New Jersey.

Attention organizations, certified personal trainers and schools:

Quantity discounts are available on bulk purchases of this publication for educational purposes or fund-raising. Special publications or publication excerpts can also be created to fit specific needs. For information, contact askROCCO Media™, 8022 South Rainbow Blvd, Suite 219, Las Vegas, NV 89139 or call 702.708.2847

Many of the following excerpts are from askROCCO columns published in either CiN Weekly, Cincinnati, OH and Juice Weekly, Des Moines, IA, both owned by Gannett Publishing.

- My personal trainer demanded I stop smoking
- Stretching before "Cardio"

Can You Believe They Asked Me This? - 69

- Can I re-center my "Headlights"?
- Should I stop having sex to gain weight?
- Is my "Unit" in trouble? Boxers or Briefs?
- Exercising your triceps can be a real "Turn On"
- I dealt with being raped at 14...
- Will people burn more fat if they strength train first?
- I'm a skinny piece of shit. How can I gain weight?
- My husband loves my "Assets." How do I get him to back off?

Dumbbells... and Treadmills... and Rubber Bands... Oh My! - 82

- Just give me the Algebra; I'll do the math myself!
- What is an E-Z Bar French Press?
- When using Nautilus machines...
- Use the equipment you have, forget the gym membership
- What you're doing on the treadmill is called "Interval Training"
- What's the difference between "Aerobic" and "Fat Burning"?
- What is the best Elliptical trainer for the buck?

I'm No Doctor and I Don't Play One on T.V. (and exercising before and after injury) - 96

- Good thing I had my trusty crystal ball
- My self-diagnosis is "fatigue disease"
- Should I follow my Doctor's advice?
- Gaining weight after Gastric Bypass
- My skin isn't bouncing back
- My knees are making creaking noises...
- I think your Doctor would agree
- Bad back… Blood thinners... what else?
- Runners and heavy objects don't mix!
- I don't want to die at an early age...
- I have a hard time exercising with Hypoglycemia
- What can I do at the gym with a broken foot?
- Coming back from Cardiac surgery
- You have to be f**kin' kidding me!

Kids Make the Fattest Moms - 121

- When to pursue a Tummy Tuck
- Desperately seeking reason
- Can't seem to get motivated after having three kids
- My whole life I've been itty-bitty
- They're a little saggy to say the least
- Fill the "Booty" bag
- You can lose 1.3 pounds a week safely
- You don't like looking like a "*marsupial*"?

I'm Still Fat After Training All These Years - 136

- If it doesn't learn, it will never burn
- I might as well be a fortuneteller
- Swimming: The worst exercise for fat loss
- I hear the word "Core"…
- Walking on the treadmill seems dreadfully boring
- Walking 60 minutes a day not enough time?

Someone Forgot to Tell You Fitness Is Free - 146

- Working out the same time every day
- Don't tell my clients or I'll be eating… cat food!
- So many books, videos, magazines… it's a bit overwhelming!
- Education is the key to motivation
- Even if you drank the "Kool Aid," it's not too late!
- My gym doesn't have a chin-up bar
- I can't afford to go to the gym
- Is there a reason you're planning for rough times?
- Should I consult a Personal Trainer?

INTRODUCTION

Controversy is nothing new to the field of health and wellness. For over thirty years I have called it as I see it — as a personal trainer to athletes, executives, beauty queens and moms, as well as an outspoken advocate for consumer common sense. Whether I answer your questions on the radio, in my weekly askROCCO™ column, askROCCO™ T.V segments, training personal trainers or conducting askROCCO™ Live events across the country, I will always give you something you can use: Real, straightforward fitness answers. I hope my mix of anecdote and irreverent candor has created a dialogue between the fat and unfat, the fit and unfit and anyone else who reads my column. Here are some observations I have noticed as I have answered your questions:

- There will always be controversy when a standard for fitness is not articulated, especially when it comes to weight training. There will always be two camps out there that will believe that they're absolutely right even though both types of training work. The goal in weight training is to promote hypertrophy (building) of muscle. Multiple sets versus lower sets and higher intensity still have the same end result: the building of muscle, except one gets you out of the gym faster. If you guessed it's the lower sets higher intensity one, you guessed right!

- Women who get pregnant and eat like they have two heads will invariably e-mail me and tell me their whole life story in three paragraphs and ask what my opinion is on why they stayed fat after the pregnancy. When I write about it in my column I will get 50-100 emails telling me what a bastard I am for saying those horrible things. Sorry ladies, but you're really not eating for two; you're eating for an embryo and you. So when you're thinking about eating that half a cheesecake and pints of ice cream with pickles, remember it all goes to your ass.
- Since the inception of this column, most of the people who went on the Atkins diet have gained their weight back and then some. All those Atkins-friendly restaurants wasted a whole lot of money to market no-carb sandwiches and meals to people who don't want to cook their own meals. The reality is if you make or cook your meals it will be much cheaper and you will almost always be eating healthier, (unless you're cooking mac & cheese every night). It is not that hard to get more fruits and vegetables into your diet AND OH MY GOSH they are carbohydrates and they are full of those crazy anti-oxidants that beat up free radicals and stop all kinds of problems as we age. Eat your damn fruits and vegetables and if you can't eat enough of them, juice them.
- Take a look around you and count how many fat people there are in your office (don't worry if you're one of them, include yourself in the mix too); that's a lot of fat people. Just think if all those fat people exercised just a little, you would have way less stress, more productivity and happier, less sick offices. Basically, a little exercise will go a long way! Do me a small favor, people in the Human Resources world, see who is fat and count the days they're out

sick, and then compare that to the people that smoke and then the people who seem relatively fit. I'd love for you to send me that data.

- Last but not least, former athletes need to stop consuming the calories they did in college or high school. Most of us ate between 4000-5000 calories when we played sports, especially the three-sport people. We were so used to eating big portions that we carried it over into our adult life. Stop it right now! And cut your portions in half; don't worry if you eat your veggies and fruits, you'll get all the nutrition you need and you won't have to eat so much of the other crap. And former athletes should also start doing something we used to do all the time: DRINK FRIGGIN' WATER. At least 1/3 of your body weight in ounces and if you want to go crazy ½ your body weight in ounces.

I want to thank my many readers and hope that my column is at the very least entertaining. Hopefully you get something out of it. I love writing this column and although it can be somewhat laborious reading all the questions you write in, please keep them coming! Don't ever forget that fitness is always free and education is the key to motivation. Read on for what I consider some of the best, worst and totally outrageous questions I've been asked and the answers I gave.

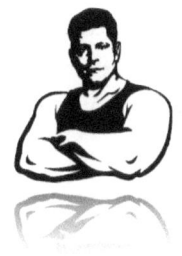

Baby wants
Back!... Arms!... Chest!... Legs!

It's very rare to have a svelte body and flabby arms.

Question: I would like a routine that will get my triceps and biceps nice and firm. I really would like to show off my arms this summer, but the way I look now I will be wearing long-sleeve garments. Please help!!
~ *Pam*

Answer: First I have to ask, is the rest of you nice and firm? Because if it isn't, your arms won't be, no matter what routine I give you. I wish people would be a little more specific; are your arms flabby or really skinny and you're ashamed to show rubber bands on two twigs? I have to tell you, it's very rare to have a svelte body and flabby arms. This is because your arms are auxiliary muscles and are usually worked when you perform compound movements, such as a Bench Press or Horizontal Row. So let's say, and I'm guessing here, your arms are flabby. I hope I guessed right because you're getting the flabby arms workout. I like people to use their own bodyweight so here's two all-around good upper body exercises that will get your arms slim and trim for the summer.

    First: Negative Pushups: Start yourself off in an up Push up position (not the wussy modified ones on your knees either), now lower yourself on a six count, 1...2...3...4...5...6, then bend your knees and raise yourself back to the up position and straighten your legs, and repeat the repetition again for 20 repetitions. Your triceps should burn and when you're finished whining

5

you can do Negative Pull-ups: You need a pull-up bar or a broomstick and two chairs for this one. If you have a pull-up bar, stand on a chair and hold on to the bar with your palms facing you, hopefully your chin is above the bar (if it isn't get a bigger chair). Now, bend your knees so that your feet aren't touching the chair and lower yourself on a six count. Place your feet back on the chair and repeat until your arms burn or until twenty, whichever comes first.

I'm tired of shopping in the juniors department

Question: I recently went through a divorce and lost some weight, I have since put the weight back on but lost 2 inches in my hips. I have gone from a size 2-3 to a 1. How can I regain the inches and gain weight? I am tired of shopping in the juniors department; at my age, most clothes are not career appropriate.

~ *Tonia*

Answer: O.K., maybe I'm crazy. Well, no, we have established that already. Umm... O.K. let's start that all over. Maybe I'm not getting all the information here but what I am getting is a little confused. You lost weight because of your divorce but now you want to gain it back in your hips. I'm sorry but almost every question I get has to do with taking inches off the hips. I'm going out on a limb here so bear with me. Let's not put inches on your hips, let's put good solid muscle on your butt and your thighs because we want you back on the market looking hot! The exercise that I recommend the most is... of course "The Lunge" (25 reps the same leg), but I want you to also find about a six-floor staircase and do the stairs two at a time for 2 sets. If you go into the askROCCO archives you should find a description of Mountain Climbers. Mountain Climbers do nothing but build your butt. So do at least 2 sets for 60 seconds and you'll be out of the juniors department before long.

It's like taking a hammer to your legs for 39 miles!

Question: Two years ago I did a Breast Cancer Charity walk where I walked 26 miles one day, then 13 the next. I did well overall with the exception of my ankles. I couldn't wear anything but flip-flops for almost a week due to the swelling. I'm doing the same walk in June 2006. Any suggestions for conditioning them?
~ *Theresa*

Answer: Wow! That's some walking there, kid. The damage you did to your ankles in this charity walk was like taking a hammer to your ankles for 39 miles. The weight from your body just kept crashing down on your ankles with each step. So the first thing I would do is go to a running shoe/sneaker store (a store that has actual runners selling their shoes) and talk to someone about serious shock-absorbing walking shoes/sneakers. You haven't told me how much you weigh, but I would consider losing a bit if you are overweight before doing this walk again. I know this is an ankle question but the reality of this situation is that you need to work out not just your ankles but the whole leg. Your hips, thighs, hamstrings and calves take in all the stress of walking. If there is a weak link such as the muscles of the thigh being weak it may place undue stress on the ankle and sometimes the lower back. I would recommend doing high rep sets of lunges on the same leg somewhere in the vicinity of 45 reps for 2 sets and then do at least 2 sets of 35 reps of calf raises on a step, making sure you stretch the calf all the way down and raise all the way up. Don't be a wuss: Push through the burn, because it will burn, baby!

Sporting a classic "Bird Chest"

Question: I'm 18, a runner, and currently sporting the classic "bird" chest. What exercises would you recommend to strengthen this area? Also, since I'm so skinny, will I fill out naturally over my college years?
~ *Phil*

Answer: I'm really not sure if the "Bird Chest" is classic but I do feel for you. This is a great question, though, because most people would think that training the chest would be the most important thing to do. Not so. Training your back and building muscle in that region will help create a wider look for you and will make your chest actually "look" bigger. While you are training your back you should shy away from doing any bench presses (with a straight bar) and do much of your work with dumbbells. Your back workout should consist of 2 sets until failure of pull-ups. If pull-ups are too hard at this point, wide grip lat pull-downs will suffice (2 sets 20 reps) some sort of horizontal row (either cable or machine) 2 sets 20 reps. For your chest, 2 sets 20 reps dumbbell press (keeping the weight over your nose), and dumbbell flyes for 2 sets of 15. To answer your second question: I'm not sure how your genetic makeup is, but usually before you hit twenty-five you will have filled out. Take a look at your father and see if he still has a "bird chest"; if he does then you'll probably have one too. Just keep training and at least you'll have a stronger better-looking "Bird Chest" then you did before.

And the questions they keepa comin'.

Question: Ok Rockhead. Since I'm so stupid, why don't you enlighten me and my "let me be a wussy" workout regime, per your "A little note for stupid people" column. This is what I want, to get big. Not big, but BIG. Currently my max on squats/dead lifts/bench is at 350/315/275. I want my bench up. I want to be able to do 315 for 5 or 6 reps easily. This is my current 4-day workout routing with reps listed for each set, excluding warm-ups. Legs: Squats 10/8/6/4, Leg press 15/12/10/10, Leg ext 4x15, Leg curl 4x15, Calves 4x15 Shoulders: Clean and press 10/8/6/4, Seated military 10/8/6/4, seated db military 10/8/6/4, rear delt flyes 4x10, shrugs 3x10 Chest: Incline 10/8/6/4, Flat 10/8/6/4, Flyes 10/8/6/4, Dips 3x15, pullovers 3x15 Back: Deads 10/8/6/4, 50 pull-ups, T-bar row 10/8/6/4, close grip row 10/8/6/4 Bi's (with chest): barbell curl 10/8/6/4, seated incline dumbbell curl 10/8/6/4 Tri's (with back or legs): close grip bench 12/10/8/6, skulls 10/8/6/4, 1 arm overhead ext 3x10, I'll switch the manner in which I lift every 3rd week (eg. switch barbell with dumbbell, or use a machine where appropriate), and on the 4th week I'll change the order of the muscle group (e.g. legs on Monday instead of chest) for another 3 weeks and the cycle repeats. So wise one, enlighten me on how I may lift to get bigger and stronger, while avoiding the affects of atrophy, while at the same time keeping the 4-day-a-week lifting regime.

~ *Chris*

Answer: You sound like a hell of a statistician. First of all you're doing more of a power-lifting workout it sounds like to me. It can and will make you stronger when doing short rep ranges. For you to gain size, oh stupid one, you need to recruit more muscle fibers. The more muscle fibers that you recruit, the more that have the capacity to grow. You are not doing that. And you're wasting an awful lot of time doing nothing that is going to get you big. If you want to get big you need to up the rep ranges for everything; the 10/8/6/4 thing is stupid and a waste of fucking time. Since you're so strong and so big try doing a rep range of 15 to twenty reps with the same weight as you do the set of 10, with a partner of course. Throw some forced reps in and a couple of negative reps and when you're done puking then e-mail me back.

Reply to answer:

Thanks for replying to my email, but I still have a couple of questions:

1. I misspoke earlier; let me clarify my main goal: to get a big bench. I've been sticking with the 10/8/6/4 rep range for a while and it has improved my bench from approximately 245 in early June to 275 in late November. I do understand the concept of recruiting more muscle fibers because I perform drop sets regularly, but won't changing my rep ranges like that work for more of an endurance or fat-burning routine?

2. With goals such as mine to be stronger and bigger (in not only bench, but everything else as well), how would I avoid atrophy and incorporate that into the muscle groups that I exercise on certain days of the week?

3. Also, should I change my rep ranges on squats, leg press, clean and press, seated military, incline, deadlift, etc. to all sets of 15?

Thank you,
~ **Chris**
(Did you notice the change of tone?)

Reply to his reply: I have nothing against what you're doing now but you do need to change up the rep ranges in order to shock the body. It's obvious to me you've hit a plateau. I would change up for about 3-4 weeks and then go back to what you were doing. From my experience, the best way to get a big bench is to perform negative sets. Take your max for the four rep sets and add 20 % more weight on the bar and lower the bar at a six-second pace. Let your training partner lift it back up and lower it again for a six; try this for 12 reps. It's impossible to not get stronger. Hope this helps.

Stop making fitness so damn complicated.

Question: I have been doing squats and lunges thinking these would help me reduce my thighs and butt. I read somewhere that this is good for "lifting" the butt area. I want to lose weight and to me, thought it would be better to lose before firming, but I do see an improvement as far as firming is concerned. My problem is how do I reduce? I've heard that the more muscle you have, the more calories you'll burn. I've been working out with free weights for the upper body and am having the same problem. I heard that less weight more reps is more for defining, versus heavy weight, less reps is for increasing. I'm confused and would greatly appreciate your expert opinion.

~ Kim

Answer: You're making me friggin' dizzy with this question, and the process that you are trying to describe is not as complicated as in your description. I think we can all take a lesson from this question. And that lesson is: STOP MAKING FITNESS SO DAMN COMPLICATED. The only things that can reduce fat on any part, and let me repeat that, ANY PART of your body is exercises that utilize fat as a fuel. So basically targeted exercises like squats and lunges will not reduce the specific fat on your ass and thighs; rather it will reduce fat elsewhere. You cannot spot reduce. Running, cycling, elliptical and even running stairs (if you don't have bad knees) will reduce fat on every part of your body, especially if done in an interval style of training.

I know this may sound absolutely foreign to you, but your body is telling you something, and that something is you need to gain muscle before it will allow you to lose fat. This is actually a good thing for you. Yes, the more muscle you have on your body the more fat calories you will expend (between 45 – 75kcals for every added pound of muscle). Talk about residual effect.

Let's talk about the fallacy and ultimate nightmare that I have been living in since I began lifting weights and exercising. The nightmare is the assumption that less weight more reps is for defining muscles and heavy weight with lower reps is for gaining muscle. I just want to scream...arghhh. Stupid people! It just doesn't happen that way. "Definition" is not just the burning of fat; it is also the building of muscle. If you build muscle you literally define it and it becomes more pronounced. Some idiot decided and wrote it down in an article and then in a book that the lower rep ranges that power lifters use would gain muscle very much like the muscle that said power lifters had. The only problem with that theory is that only a small percentage of the population has that much fast twitch muscle fiber to acclimate their bodies to that kind of program. But of course if it's written down then it must be gospel. If you were to truly work out like that you would have to do a million sets to break down the muscle adequately. Remember: Build muscle first and the fat will fall off.

Eating right and aerobic exercise won't keep your belly flat.

Question: First of all, you're awesome!! I was training with a trainer at my local gym and stopped eventually because I didn't want to bulk up. He's a great trainer, but bodybuilders' bods are what are beautiful to him. I want to remain feminine.

So, I have been going to the gym 3 times a week for 25 minutes on the Elliptical machine. I walk for 2 minutes, run for 3 minutes for the entire 25 minutes, and then cool down. I eat yogurt for breakfast, chicken breast & veggies for lunch, a light and healthy dinner. Eating badly has never been my problem. I drink a gallon of water a day...very aware of what I put in my body. What though else can I do to tone my abs... or lack of? The sit-up machines @ the gym? Crunches? Please help. I want to look fabulous in my bikini.

Keep up the great work,

~ Carly

Answer: Thank you for the kind words. I'm not so sure I'm going to have kind words for you because I think you're doing yourself a disservice by not keeping up with at least a maintenance strength-training workout. I have to tell you that just eating right and aerobic exercise isn't going to make your belly flat or lose the fat on it. Your midsection is composed of three main muscle groups and they all interact with each other. If one is lacking then the others suffer also. The contour (shape) of your "abs" depends solely on the amount of muscle you have. Imagine wanting to sculpt a figure out of clay but there is no clay to be had. It would be quite impossible to sculpt that figure. Without muscle (clay) you can't provide shape, and that shape includes flatness. I'm not a big fan of ab machines in the gym only because they sometimes cause people to work in an unnatural way. Working your abdominal area with crunches that bring your upper body off the ground, crisscross crunches, and practicing flexing your abdomen are really all you need to do to keep the belly flat and contoured. Hopefully this will get you into that bikini you're looking forward to getting!

All my weight goes to my back. What can I do?

Question: Please help me... I don't have any idea what exercise to do to burn the fat off my back. I have a cone shape. All my weight goes to my back. What can I do? Thank you.
~ *Laura*

Answer: You're question is probably the second most asked question next to "How do I get rid of my butt?" The reason you accumulate fat on your back is because there is usually no muscle there to fill your skin, so fat decides to move in. If you develop some back muscle you will see that the muscle will kick the fat's ass and throw it out. Some great back exercises that no one does anymore are Jumping Jacks (at least 50), a few others that people still do are: Horizontal row (on a machine), Lat Pulldown (also on a machine). Developing muscle in your back will also help even out that cone shape you have.

Senior citizens need firm arms too!

Question: How can I tone and firm my arms. I am a senior citizen and my arms keep waving even after I've stopped.
~ *Sue*

Answer: I'm glad to see there's a senior citizen reading askROCCO. I guess it's true people do believe I can help people from 8 to 80. One question to you though, why does everyone that supposes to be a senior citizen always ask me how to firm up their arms? I would think that by the time you got to be your age you would have figured it out. Maybe not. Flabby arms do suck! When you're waving good-bye and your arm keeps waving long after you're gone... oooh, that's a dilemma! Now that you want to beat me with a switch I'll answer your question. First you need to fill the empty bags that are your arms. Over the years you let your muscles atrophy (melt away); but not to worry, research has shown that no matter what age you start training you will build muscle. Maybe not as fast as an eighteen-year–old, but you can. First, take an empty half-gallon jug you bought from Kroger (do you like how I'm fishing for endorsement opportunities?) and fill it with enough water that you can lift performing a tricep press: With one arm reach over your head holding the jug, and slowly bend your elbow (obviously in a descending motion). When your elbow breaks parallel to the floor then raise it up again. Perform this 15 times then switch to the other arm. Now take the same jug and stand up straight with your arm to the side and raise it (keeping your elbow pointing down) so that the jug touches your bicep and perform these 15 times also. If you have dumbbells on hand you can also use them, but don't buy them if you don't have to.

Help! I'm getting arms like my mother.

Question: Help! I'm getting arms like my mother. I am looking for exercises to build up my arms. I have 1-lb, 3-lb & 5-lb weights at home along with a newly purchased exercise rubber band. Are there exercises that I can do with the equipment that I own? Thanks.
~ Susan H

Answer: Obviously, "arms like your mother" is a bad thing. I'm thinking. They probably keep waving long after she's stopped. Lots of loose skin and fat, yeah, that pretty much sucks. Well, the first thing I would do is throw that stupid exercise band in the garbage. Here's my problem with exercise bands: They don't work. Really! There is something called a strength curve within your range of motion around a specific joint. Usually when you provide resistance, in this case an exercise band, most of your strength is needed at the beginning and middle of the movement, with strength tapering towards the end of that movement. Exercise bands give no resistance at the beginning, medium resistance in the middle with a whole lot of tension at the top of the movement. Common sense will usually tell anyone that this seems a little backwards, BECAUSE IT IS! Idiotic trainers thought this would be a fun and fulfilling way to train people. Well it's not. Physical therapists use bands when there is barely any strength in the muscle. What was the other question? That's right, exercises you can do at home. Yes there is. Thank you and have a nice day. Oh, oh, you wanted me to tell you. Bicep curls: While sitting in a chair facing a mirror, place your arms at your sides with your palms facing the mirror, keeping your shoulders back and head up, bend your elbow and raise your arm towards your shoulder, and slowly lower it. I've given enough great advice; you'll have to wait for another article for the tricep press. I think I'm out of room.

Upper-body strength for Wakeboarding

Question: Dear Rocco, I'm a petite 108-lb. 30-something female that enjoys water sports. I've been wakeboarding for the past three years. I enjoy it tremendously and I am always looking to improve. (Wakeboarding is similar to water skiing except you're on a small board instead of skis.) Here's my problem. Wakeboarding requires a lot of upper-body strength. And you guessed it: I have none or very little. I've been told that if I can develop my upper back and shoulder strength, I will gain better control of the rope and handle making me a better boarder. Since last fall I've been doing a combination of running or jogging and weight lifting about three to four times a week. Do you have any recommended exercises that will target my shoulders and upper back and help me increase my strength in those areas?

~ Water lover

Answer: I'm so glad you cleared up that Wakeboarding term. I don't know what I would've done (maybe watch ESPN2 for more exciting Extreme Game stuff). Maybe you can help me understand that curling thing next; or actually, maybe not. Here's the short answer to your question. Although the Extreme Sports experts that clued you in to needing upper body strength probably were right, one thing needs to be said. Without a good foundation you're building your house on sand. For those who can't read between the lines I'll explain: You need to have strong legs before you can build your upper body. This will help provide symmetry and make you become much stronger. Now to help with the upper body exercises; any exercise that simulates a rowing motion such as a Horizontal Row, Floor Pulley or actual rowing machine would probably help greatly. Without seeing you in person I can't recommend too much more except for good abdominal work that includes exercises that work the external obliques. (Medicine ball twists are a good start.) Good luck and Hang Ten or whatever you dudes and dudettes say anymore.

I'd love to be like Hillary Swank.

Question: I'm a 5'3 125-lb female and would love to be like Hillary Swank and work out to sweat hard. Only issue is that I am super sore after lifting weights. I practice everything you preach (as a Rocco-follower should) and recently increased my weight training to 2 sets of 20, increased the amount of weight I lift to burn more fat, and do cardio after I lift to ensure even more fat burning.

A couple of questions... How often should I work out the same muscle groups? Every couple of days or whenever the soreness goes away?

Also, is there one muscle group you would recommend I train harder to look my best?

Thanks!

~ *L.K.*

Answer: Hey L.K. we don't have to be so secretive with our identity; I'm not giving out your social security number or anything. I love to hear that you're working out hard and at least say you're following what I write. There are a couple of theories on this question. I will give you mine first; soreness is an indication that lactic acid is present and that you may have over-trained that muscle or muscle group. This is my opinion only, there is no documentation or research to prove or disprove this but I would rather wait until the soreness goes away if you are working out that hard. Your body needs more rest than exercise when you train at higher intensities. Now the other side of that coin says that in order to get the lactic acid out of the area you need to exercise. I'm not a big fan of over-training so I only train twice a week on Monday and Thursday because I'm usually sore for two days and then I can hit it hard again Thursday. You may notice that at the beginning of the week you can go crazy hard but the energy wanes towards the end of the week if you're trying to go hard four or six times a week training. Keep training hard and hope to see some photos of that hard body in some fitness magazine.

You're fit, you're healthy, now shut up!

Question: Muscle feels good. I never thought that I would want to lose muscle mass, but recently I have considered trying to taper down. Years and years of swimming have provided me with strong, wide, solid shoulders that make tops fit too tightly but then fit too loosely everywhere else ("nearly-A" chest size, etc.). I am 5'-7", 135 lbs. I cross-train with running, weights, swimming, yoga. Any suggestions on a change in my routine that could reduce my shoulder bulk but not compromise strength?

~ *Mary*

Answer: People always want what they don't have. That's America for you! Why would you ever want to lose muscle? That's crazy. You know what? I have a car that's been doing great for me but I think I'll take the engine out and see what happens. If you can read between the lines, that's good, if you can't, obviously it would be pretty dopey to pull the engine out of a perfectly good car now wouldn't it? So here's what I suggest. Take up sewing and start making clothes that can actually fit you. You're fit; you're healthy, now shut up.

Well I've thought it over and I think you would be better off eliminating actual shoulder movements from your workout. Your shoulder joint is used almost too much in many workouts. If you're doing flyes keep doing them, eliminate pressing from the bench, and keep any rowing movements. These exercises work the shoulder joint at an auxiliary level and won't compromise strength.

How can I get "quick flat abs"?

Question: I have a question for you. How would I get quick flat abs? I have been trying for so long.
Thank You.
~ *Samantha*

Answer: There are many ways to answer this question. First, if you've been trying for so long, why did it take you this long to ask me this question? Second, you need to give me a little more information. Look, if you're three hundred pounds, nothing I tell you will get you flat abs quickly. Even if you're fifteen pounds overweight you can't quickly get your abs flat. Let's say that you're at your right weight, and have been doing sit-ups or crunches for a long time, but you still have a protruding belly. This happens when you build up too much muscle in the center part of your midsection, (the rectus abodominus) which is usually referred to as the six pack, even though there are eight sections to it. Without working the outer muscles, (the external obliques) the six pack muscles tend to protrude way past any place that you want them to.

Now if you are fat, you need to lean out a bit before I can give you more advice. Just to humor you though, since you gave me so much to go on here, I'll give you my favorite exercise for making the abs flat. It's called a crisscross crunch and can be done several ways but I'm only going to tell you two of them.

Lay flat on your back facing up and place the soles of your feet on a wall of some kind (don't wear your sneakers, because you'll wind up asking me to re-paint

27

your wall, and trust me I'm not doing it), and place your hands behind your head and keep your elbows flat. While keeping your elbows flat, raise your left elbow to the outside of your right knee and come back down slowly. Then, bring your right elbow to the outside of your left knee and come down slowly again. Now Simon says do as many as you can without having a heart attack. I said I was going to give you two examples, well I lied. Actually, place your feet on a chair and now you have another option. Hope you get those "quick flat abs" that you've wanted for so long.

Gaining size in the "Glutes"?

Question: What are the best exercises for working the glutes? I want to gain size not reduce. How many sets, reps, etc.? I am currently only doing a leg/glute workout once a week. Since I want to gain mass is 1x a week ideal?

~ Cathy

Answer: This is great! Most of the time women write to me wanting to get rid of their booty and you want to get one. I love it. You know what, I think I should give a "How to Get a Booty Clinic" because many Cincinnati women don't have any backsides to speak of and if they do have one it's usually flat and wide.

Now that I've alienated all my women readers with no butts, I'll answer your question. You need to work your legs and glutes three times a week with higher repetition ranges. Not those stupid bodybuilder four sets of ten leg workouts. You need to recruit as many muscle fibers as you can. The higher repetition ranges will do just that. I recommend one set of lunges for 30-35 repetitions on the same leg (do not alternate!) one set of Mountain Climbers for 60 seconds (if you don't know what a Mountain Climber is, corner the nearest football coach) then do one more set of 25-30 Lunges and another set of Mountain Climbers for 60 seconds. Do this on a consistent basis and you'll have the booty you've always dreamed of.

A guaranteed way to get rid of "Love Handles"

Question: Hi Rocco, I am sure you've heard this question a million times before. I would like to know if there is any guaranteed way to get rid of love handles. It really bothers me now, I have my whole body in really good shape, almost no fat anywhere except on the side if my stomach. I can even see my six-pack now but still there are those bad love handles. I would do anything to get rid of them. Thanks.
~ *Jiri*

Answer: Actually, I've heard this question a million and one times, but who am I to count. I do have to ask you a question though, doesn't it suck not having askROCCO™ down in Louisville? I heard there's a nice little weekly there called Velocity just itching for quality fitness & exercise advice. Maybe they'll call...but maybe Louisville likes their people to look like their horses; it's Derby time you know. I'm sure they'll call now!

You, like a million other people, try so desperately to take something away from your body such as love handles, but you don't get the point. The reason why there's fat hanging down on your sides is because you need to fill that area with something, preferably muscle. When we're younger our body has some kind of balance, as we age some of the muscle that we used for sports or activity gets lost somewhere between college and actually working for a living. The best way to get rid of love handles is to fill the bag, not throw the bag out. Translated, that means you must add muscle to the area and gravity can't wreak havoc. Try some crisscross crunches: lying on the floor face up, knees bent; Sit up with your hands behind your head and arms flat, bring your left elbow just past your right knee, then alternate until you can't do any more.

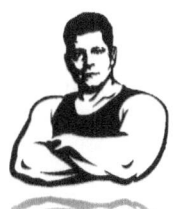

When "Good" Diets Go "Bad"

You're just like millions of Americans that don't listen.

Question: I've recently lost weight on a sensible diet. Now I've incorporated weight training 4 times a week along with 6-day-a-week cardio. How many calories should I be eating to continue the weight loss, but maximize my workouts? Please break this down into protein/carbs/fat too.
~ Kelly

Answer: Well, Kelly you've already screwed up. You've decided to lose weight on a diet and although it is sensible, without resistance exercise in the mix you've definitely lost lean mass or muscle weight and this is bad. Don't worry, though, you're just like the millions of other Americans that don't listen. You need to begin an exercise program first before you think about a healthy eating schedule. I know I'm going to get hundreds of e-mails from dietitians saying that eating right is just as important, but it is too hard to focus on two things at the same time, especially dieting. Once you've begun an exercise program that fits your lifestyle and has become part of that lifestyle, then and only then do I recommend adding eating sensibly as part of the equation.

Most people fail because they don't understand this. Jack La Lanne told me at a conference once, *"I've seen more unhealthy people who eat right and don't exercise, than people who exercise and don't eat right."* I agree with him. With what you told me about the frequency of the workout, I think you're overdoing it a bit. Try to do a full-body workout three days a week and if you think you need more aerobic exercise then do it in between your workouts. If you do too much, burnout is very likely. If you're eating sensibly like you said I wouldn't worry too much about the eating part. But if you are a worrier, I won't help you with the diet part; I'm not licensed for that. Go talk to a dietician, because most of the time good advice isn't free.

I think you'll tell me the truth

Question: A friend of mine is on the Atkins diet and has lost a lot of weight. I'm thinking about going on it but wanted your opinion first. You seem to tell it like it is and I think you'll tell me the truth.
~ *Mindy*

Answer: I'm not a dietician and don't ever claim to be. But if you want my opinion I'll give it to you. If I hear one more word about the Atkins diet I'm going to dig that idiot up and beat the living daylights out of him. Anyone who believes they can promote a diet that leaves a whole food group out of your eating equation is at minimum, high and at most just plain stupid. I don't care if he was a doctor or not. Ketosis, if you do any research, is never a good thing. It's actually a very dangerous state for your body to be in. Even if Atkins had purported to have 25,000 patients go through his program unscathed. He must've been Super Doctor to attend to all those people. But why do any research on your own, the Atkins marketing machine has done it for you, hasn't it? So let your friend keep sucking in bacon by the pound and call me when you need my jackhammer to unclog her arteries.

How many calories per day should I consume?

Question: Good Morning!
I am 5'5" and I weigh 130. I do strength training 3 times a week and intensive cardio 5 times a week. I love to exercise! This is not the problem. I AM UNSURE HOW MANY CALORIES PER DAY I SHOULD TAKE IN. I don't want to be "bone thin" but I would like to look leaner. I would like to lose 5 more pounds of fat (because I have a body fat % of 20 and fat mass of 25lbs). I have tried dropping down to 1200 cals and I had no energy; I didn't feel I was feeding my body what it needed. Another trainer told me 1600 and I gained weight. PLEASE HELP!
~ Karen

Answer: Help is on the way! Whoever that trainer was who told you to take in only 1600 kcals is an idiot and should be slapped upside his head. The reason why you gained weight is because your body was starving and didn't know what else to do when you put 400 more calories into it. Here's a news flash! You cannot starve fat off your body. Fat is fuel and needs to be burned off. The weight that you lose when you starve yourself is muscle weight and when you begin to put nourishment back into your body the muscle wants to come back, and it will if you're working out. The stupidity of some trainers never ceases to amaze me. The reality of your situation is that you should have been taking in 2313 kcals just to keep your body fueled for the exercise you told me you were doing. Stay consistent with your workout; maybe up the intensity just a bit and stay away from sugar and you'll drop that body fat. If you love exercise then the consistency shouldn't be a problem. Good luck.

Do it yourself Liposuction?

Question: Hey Rocco! Please help this fat girl! I am 6 ft tall I have lost about 20 lbs altogether since May. I can't get past 273 lbs. I am eating right; I exercise 4-5 times per week. I do weights and abs 2 times per week, the elliptical for 50 to 57 minutes 3 times per week. I do the leg lifts lying on the floor and on the other thing where I lift my legs from a standing position. I eat breakfast, take vitamins... What am I doing wrong?! It's frustrating me! Please help me or I will have to do my own liposuction and cut off the excess skin with a butcher knife!

~ Queenla

Answer: O.K., Queenla, quit with the do-it-yourself liposuction! Butcher knives are not that sharp and the scarring would not be pretty. You do have a dilemma though. I hear this so much I think I'm going to write a book called "I've lost twenty pounds and can't go any more." This is so common that it's almost comical, except in your case it pretty much sucks. Here's the problem. At almost 300 lbs your body had the opportunity to lose weight and 20 lbs is the easiest to lose. Many times as we go on this journey called body re-discovery the weight and fat comes off in twenty-pound increments. If it comes off too quickly your body will re-regulate itself because in most cases the weight that came off had muscle attached to it. Once the body re-regulates itself you will have the opportunity again to burn more fat. You need to realize that your body can only burn between 1.3 and 2 lbs successfully and safely; any more is muscle. If you do the math correctly that would be 67.6 lbs on the low side and an almost impossible 104 lbs on the high side.

38

I believe your intensity and your frequency may be your biggest problem. I would increase your weight training to three times per week with some interval aerobic training on your weight training days even if for only 15 – 20 minutes. On the other days walk two minutes at a good clip and than raise the incline to 5% or higher. This style of training will create chaos in your energy burning systems of the body. Stay the course, don't get discouraged and you'll be svelte in no time.

Eat before or after your workout?

Question: Is it better to eat before or after working out? My fiancé and I get home from work around 4:30 and don't know if we should eat a meal and then head to the gym or head straight to the gym and eat after.
~*Jennifer*

Answer: When do you eat lunch? If you follow a five- to six-meal sensible eating plan then you should eat a small snack at about 3:00pm; that should be sufficient to hold you through the workout. More importantly you use the food you ate the day before as your energy source today because your body stores the complex carbohydrates as glycogen in your liver and muscles to help you perform your exercise movements. I personally like to have something light in my stomach before I work out but it's different for everyone. However after every workout you should get some really good carbs into your body within the first 30 minutes after your workout. By good carbs I mean fruits like melons, apples, oranges and vegetables (salads are the easiest). Replenishing your body with these foods will help in the energy and muscle reparation process. Keep up the workout; you're doing more than 65% of Cincinnatians are. I just wish more people would get off their ass and at least try something.

Don't do something half-assed

Question: I have always exercised and tried to eat healthy, although I do have a weakness for sweets and pizza. I still eat those foods, I just make sure to eat healthy most of the time and stay active. I have always been against diets, because like you I don't believe they work. However, lately I have had a hard time sticking to healthy eating. I seem to crave sweets more than usual, and have a hard time sticking to healthy portions of them. I'm 30 now, and I can tell a difference between now and just a few years ago. I have 2 children, and I had no problem losing the baby weight. It's just becoming more difficult to eat healthy. I'm a single mom, work full time, plus my kids play sports year round. With our hectic lifestyle I need food that is quick and easy to prepare. My company has a gym, so I work out on my lunch break. I would like some tips on controlling cravings and being healthier for myself and my children.

~ Heather

Answer: First I'm going to tell you that you are the parent and that your kids shouldn't run your life. Many of us create hectic lifestyles and chaos just to give our life some semblance of meaning. We tend to place too much stress on ourselves to make excuses why we don't have time to do what's right in our lives. Priorities need to be set. If you're not providing good nutrition for you or your children, then neither one of you will be as productive as you need to be and being so busy really doesn't mean squat when you're not able to do it right. If you do something half-assed you'll always produce a half-assed outcome. With that said, stress is a major cause of creating an insatiable appetite for sweets and other sugary items. The more stress you heap on yourself the more sweets you crave. Take a look at what may be causing you stress. Try not to keep sweets around because if there's access to them then you may crave them more. Once you start down that road your brain can't seem to shut itself off. Stay away from artificial sweeteners because they will make you crave sweets even more. Another issue is that sugar, specifically, hits a part of the brain that provides a sense of satisfaction, and is often used as a substitute for the lack of sex, lack of communication and emotions. I'm not a psychologist and will never claim to be, lord knows I need my share of therapy. So take this as one man's opinion backed with some experience. One important note is to make sure you don't totally deprive yourself of anything because that will drive you to crave or even obsess over it.

It is a big step for me

Question: I am ready to start working out and eating better. I have taken the initiative to get a membership at a gym, but nutritionally I need some help also. Would you recommend a nutritionist or a dietician to help me learn what to eat and how to eat to achieve a healthier lifestyle? Right now, I have only been able to walk on the treadmill for 20 minutes and then I have to go home because I am so beat. I do this every day and have now done it for the last 20 days. It is a big step for me, but, little by little, things will increase and I will be healthier. Can you give a beginner any insight though? Thanks.
~ **Michelle,** *Omaha, Nebraska*

Answer: Yes, I can give you advice; I can always give advice. If you heed the advice is another matter. Let's say you will. If you are fat then I wouldn't recommend walking on the treadmill right now; I would rather you begin a strength-training program that involves all the muscle groups of your body concentrating on the legs for now. You need to build muscle in the legs to help in shock absorption for aerobic activity. Perform all the strength training first with an eight-minute warm-up in the beginning and increase your aerobics in small increments. Now I have to ask you a question, what the hell are you doing in Omaha, Nebraska? I always heard that there are only two things in Omaha... Steers and Queers, and you don't sound like any of them. I just had to say that. I think I'm the only guy that loved that movie. Well, good luck with the advice.

Does anyone care that some people want to gain weight?

Question: I have noticed all these low-carb diets, lose-weight plans, etc. lately. Does anyone care that maybe some people want to gain weight? Some do, so I actually ask co-workers what they are being told to lose weight and I do that but it's not working. Are there any weight-gain pills, plans, or advice you can offer? (I am serious about people trying to gain weight.)
~ *Tonya, Cincinnati via New Jersey*

Answer: I don't know why you would ask co-workers what they do to lose weight if you want to gain weight. Are you trying reverse psychology on yourself? To answer your question: yes there are ways to gain weight. The only real weight that you should really care about gaining is muscle weight. It is unhealthy to want to gain fat weight. If you're consistent with a sensible strength-training program and consume at least 50-60 % of your diet in carbohydrates you will gain muscle. Carbohydrates do something called "protein sparing." So you use the carbohydrates for energy and not protein (as with the low-carb diets). This enables you to gain muscle faster. And NO! Protein shakes are not a good way to gain weight. Food, real food is a good way to get your nourishment. So to wrap this up, eat more carbohydrates and strength train and as those cartoons of Charles Atlas in the back of Boys Life say: You won't be a 90-lb weakling anymore.

Get off the damn "Atkins Diet"!

Question: I've been on the Atkins diet since April 2004 and have lost 27 pounds. I've not lost an ounce since early November. I'm considering changing to a low-fat/calorie diet. My fear is that I will begin to gain once I add carbs back into my diet. My goal is 15 to 20 pounds more. I also work out at Curves 5 days a week and ride an exercise bike at home. Any advice or suggestions would be appreciated. Thanks for your time.
~ *Terri*

Answer: Get off the damn Atkins diet; obviously it stopped working and you hit a huge plateau. When that diet was first introduced it was actually only for people who needed to lose extreme amounts of fat fast because of some type of surgery they were going to have. Think about this: If you replace most of the protein that the idiot Atkins tells you to eat with vegetables and fruit you would be much healthier and you would have lost more weight. I'm glad he's dead; I just wish his diet books would have been buried with him. Keep up the working out but make sure that the intensity is ever increasing. Don't just go to the gym, actually work out and you'll start to see fat loss again. Be consistent with the exercise and DO NOT go on another stupid diet.

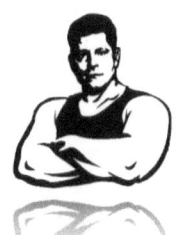

Your Trainer is an Idiot
(and other people who give stupid advice)

A fitness instructor and I were discussing this question

Question: A fitness instructor and I were discussing this question about push-ups and would like to get your thoughts. I have been going to the gym daily for more than 6 months, and combined with diet, have managed to lose 40 pounds. While ab work has gotten easier and cardio has gotten easier, and even weight work has gotten easier--forcing me to do more crunches, adding more weight, longer workouts etc., push-ups continue to be as hard as they ever were. You would figure that by losing that weight, there would be less weight to "push" and therefore would get easier. But doing my 50 push-ups feels as hard as they did on the first day. Is this a mental thing or is there some sort of explanation?

~ Robert Lee

Answer: I want to congratulate you on losing the 40 pounds; that's a pretty great accomplishment. Now that that's done, why the hell are you asking me this question if you had a fitness instructor standing right next to you? What is he getting paid for? To look good in shorts and a tank top? It's tough to find good help these days. Although I'm a little disappointed that your fitness instructor didn't know the answer I'll tell you so you can tell him. There are many factors that contribute to this problem. Usually it has to do with mechanics and muscle fiber type. I would bet that your arms are long and you have fast-twitch muscle fibers in most of your upper body muscle groups. The longer your arms are the more distance you have to cover and push against gravity. Fast-twitch muscle fibers are very explosive fibers and have a very short attention span. There may be one factor you're not considering and that may be that you're not working your back enough. The back or Lats are a stabilizer muscle to the chest and shoulders and are a very important component in developing strength. With all that said who wants to do more than 50 push-ups anyway? Place a 20-pound plate on your back and keep doing your50, just make sure the plate doesn't fall off and smack you in the head. That's all I need.

Metabolism of a dead turtle

Question: Rocco, What can you do if you're on medication that slows down your metabolism to pretty much a dead turtle? For the last 6 months, I have worked out 6 days a week... 3 days a week with a personal trainer doing weight training and 3 days a week doing cardio. I saw some improvement, but not enough to show all the work I really did. I should have been a size 6 after all the workouts and healthy eating. My trainer couldn't explain it either. I plan on going to the seminar that addresses this situation, but what can I do in the meantime?

~ Gina, California

Answer: It's nice that askROCCO reaches as far as California. I wish a paper would pick me up there but I don't think those granola-crunching, tree-hugging and earthquake-having, surfer dudes and dudettes could handle this column, but who am I to judge? I have to tell you, a dead turtle is... well dead! and doesn't have a metabolism... I think we humans still have something that resembles a metabolism even though it may not feel like it. If the medication you're taking is an SSRI (selective serotonin re-uptake inhibitor) the answer is no! There is pretty much nothing you can do about the weight gain. Some of the research that's out there suggests that the weight gain is not fat but water. The medications trigger a hormone that is considered an anti-diuretic or water-retaining hormone. The problem is no matter how much exercise you do you can't burn water. If you can't get off the medication I suggest you try to build as much muscle as you can to be able to handle the extra baggage. How much were you paying your trainer anyway? Hope to see you at the seminar.

There will always be conflicting advice.

Question: O.K., Rocco. I need some help and you're first on my list of who to ask. I'm a 250+ pound 30-something–year-old male that started working out in the gym about 3 months ago. I'm going 5 days a week, an hour or so each time, and doing a combination of weights and walking. My problem is that, after doing this exercise and eating a healthy vegetarian diet, I'm still not losing weight as quickly as I'd like. I have tried to read up and get some ideas, but one book says that the treadmill is bad because it causes your heart rate to go too high and then your body burns glucose and not fat. Another book says that a treadmill is better and burns fat faster. What gives? I don't mind putting in the effort and working as hard as I need to, but I'd like to make sure I'm spending my time wisely. My main goal is to burn fat and lose weight, so in addition to weight training to build muscle, which cardio activity is better - the treadmill or walking around the track at the gym?
Help! Ready to lose.

~ Jason

Answer: The problem is everyone and their brother has an opinion on what works and what doesn't. My opinion is that consistency and dedication is what gets results... no more, no less. Intensity, Frequency and Duration are the keys to the inner universe and now they're yours to keep. Your intensity must be high. Your frequency must be consistent (three times a week) and your duration must be succinct (do not waste time in the gym).

The easy answer to your question would be that you're not doing enough work. To give you the right answer would be that you need to create chaos in your energy systems and the best way to do that is to perform some type of interval training. If you are using the treadmill, then walk for two minutes then run for two minutes, walk for two minutes then run again for two minutes. Do this for twenty minutes or until you're ready to drop but not more then thirty minutes. You'll start to see the pounds come off. You can also do this on a track outside if you prefer, vary it up if you want. Don't worry too much about the conflicting advice. Filter what is out there, take what you can use and leave the rest for the suckers.

Prepare your body by doing

Question: My friend wants me to join him this spring on bike rides at a 15-mile-per-hour pace for 1 to 2 hours. What is the best way to get ready for this? I hate the exercise bike. I currently walk and run on a treadmill or outside when weather permits at varying speeds 4.0-4.8 mph at different inclines for 30 minutes 6 days a week. I also do some arm and leg weight machines 3 days a week to maintain my 5'3" frame at 140 pounds.
Carolyn

Answer: I've always been under the assumption that you prepare yourself for whatever you're going to do by actually doing what you're going to do. Maybe you've heard of this thing called common sense. Someone the other day told me that they started to run on the treadmill to get ready for the "Climb the Carew Tower" event and I just started shaking my head in disbelief.

So I suggested that person actually climb a couple of flights of stairs just to get a clue of what it feels like to climb stairs. I'm saying the same to you. If you don't like the exercise bike then get on a real bike and see if you even like cycling. If it's a little to cold for you to go outside then check out a local Spinning Class at your local gym. If this doesn't strike your fancy, I'm sorry but you're SOL. Just to let you in on a little secret, 15 miles an hour for one to two hours is a pretty difficult pace and if you don't enjoy cycling it can make for a very uncomfortable ride. I love cycling and that is a real pain in the ass to me... literally.

Is this normal or did my trainer overwork me?

Question: I recently joined a well-known worldwide gym. I am 39 and healthy. I have always done cardio but weight training is new to me. I worked with a personal trainer twice since joining. I did 2-3 sets of 12 for each of the exercises and told my trainer my goal was to develop more muscle tone to counteract age-related muscle loss. After both training sessions, the first for legs and abs and the second for chest and arms, I was very sore for about 3 days. The pain was so bad I had to take over-the-counter pain relievers. I could hardly walk up and down steps after the leg training and couldn't lift my arms above my shoulders after the chest/arm training. My legs were sore enough that I had to suspend my daily walking program for 2 days. Is this normal or did my trainer possibly overwork me?

~ Christine

Answer: It's obvious to me that your trainer took the phrase "no pain, no gain" literally. He or she is an idiot! What was this trainer trying to do, give you all the muscle mass you needed in two workouts? I hate these crazy workout zealots. To answer your question: no this is not normal and yes, I will say it again your trainer is an idiot. I do believe you should perform work intense enough to provide desired results and mild to medium soreness on the first couple of workouts, but to have to suspend other activities in the process is just plain stupid. Next time you see them, roll this issue of CiN Weekly up and smack them over the head with it and please make sure my picture is facing them as you continue beating them. Here's a word to my fellow colleagues: with every workout, we take our clients' lives in our hands. So don't try to kill your clients on the first workout.

Your trainer should have known better

Background: I recently started working out with a personal trainer. I'm basically in good shape EXCEPT I had not been to the gym on a regular basis for about 4 months.

Question: After 2 sessions (48 hours in between) of weight training, my left arm won't straighten out without great pain. My first workout was focused on triceps and the second back, which included working my biceps. The bend area around my elbow area is very sore and I just can't seem to get relief. Do you think I injured it?
~ Anonymous

Answer: The short answer is yes, I believe you injured yourself but since I have no medical license I highly recommend you go see someone who has one, preferably in orthopedics. Then when you can move your arm, go slap the friggin' trainer who did this to you over the head with a baseball bat. Your trainer should have known better than to train you that hard right after a long layoff like 4 months. I'm not saying he should have taken it easy on you either but your upper arm muscles or the triceps and biceps should not even be worked the first week back to training. If you work the larger muscle groups, like chest and back the auxiliary or smaller muscle groups get a workout also. There is no need in the initial workouts to isolate single joint muscles unless there are particular injuries that need special attention. I will apologize for his stupid ass because I think his pride probably won't allow him to.

An opinion on sports supplements?

Question: Hey Rocco! I was flipping through one of those workout magazines the other day, and I think 90% of it was advertisements for supplements! What's your opinion of all those sports supplements out on the market? Also, what do you think of those magazines like *Muscle & Fitness*, *Flex*, *Muscle Media*, etc.?
~ *Gavin*

Answer: Supplements, the billion-dollar industry that preys on lazy, pathetic wannabes. Supplement ads, especially in Joe Weider publications, promise you everything that a pubescent boy or girl could imagine. From big muscles to a big penis or breasts, please... Exercise, nutrition and the proper mental attitude (positive self-image) are the only things you need to lose fat permanently. Supplements are not a requirement. Some basic supplements are helpful for "nutritional insurance," and some supplements can help speed up the fat loss process *a little*, but not nearly as much as the advertising leads you to believe. Even supplements that have been proven effective are only responsible for a small fraction of the results you achieve. I believe that at least 97% of your results will come from good training and good nutrition. If most of your results come from nutrition and training, then why would you chase after that last 3% "edge" if you haven't even maximized the *first* 97%? Isn't that approach completely backwards?

Once you've reached a high level of development from intelligent, intense, methodical training and quality nutrition, and the closer you get to your ultimate genetic potential, the slower your progress will become. Progress can and will continue indefinitely, but as you reach higher levels of achievement, this is when supplements and other "minor" details make the most difference.

In world-class athletics, competitions can be won or lost by hundredths of a second, a tenth of a point, a fraction of a pound, or a single judge's opinion. The extra 3% that supplements might provide could be the difference between winning and losing.

Now look at the average beginner or intermediate: They're still eating junk foods and skipping meals. They're not even working out consistently. And what do they do FIRST? You guessed it; they immediately run out searching for a "shortcut" in the form of a pill, powder or latest diet.

It's a shame that so many people look for easy ways instead of making the effort to learn how to eat and train. I don't know if you wanted me to go on a rant, but I thought I would give you the opinion you asked for. The people at GNC probably want to put a hit out on me right now.

Settle this debate! Which burns more calories...?

Question: I've had a constant debate with a girlfriend for months over a couple fitness questions, so I'm hoping you can settle this once and for all:

1.) Which burns more calories - jogging at a constant speed or doing intervals (walk, jog fast, walk, jog fast, walk - you get the idea)?

2.) Which burns more calories - doing cardio before or after lifting weights?

Thanks in advance for your thoughtful, yet sarcastic insight! I'm looking forward to it...
~ Kimberly

Answer: Sarcastic...huh?! Insightful, yes, but sarcastic, never! Come on, is it really a debate, or is it a bet that you want me to settle? If it's a bet, then I want half of the winnings. Go on, call me greedy. If you don't like it, then call "Body by Jake." He may even have something insightful to say besides "abbadabbas."

To answer your question and settle the debate once and for all: An individual will burn more fat calories performing an interval-style aerobic workout, i.e. walk two minutes, run two minutes, walk two minutes, rinse and repeat, than they would with sustained speed training. The reason for this is that the body becomes very efficient at utilizing energy during sustained training. However, when interval training is introduced, the body doesn't know what the hell to do, so it keeps burning fat. That's the simple explanation.

To answer your second question, wait a minute, how lucky are you guys, getting two questions answered for the price of one? OK, back to business now; I've been saying this for years and I hope it finally sinks in. First, you need to do a little warm-up, nothing too crazy, just 6-8 minutes on the treadmill, elliptical trainer, bike... whatever. Then, perform a strength-training workout. After that, you should finish up with aerobic training. The workout is much more efficient this way. To illustrate my point; let's say you begin your workout with 30 minutes of aerobic training before you do your strength training. Now you've just wasted about 15 minutes, because during your first 13-17 minutes all you're burning is glycogen, which is the fuel the supplies your muscles. It's only around minute 18, that you even start to burn fat, but by now, you've already depleted much of the glycogen stores that you'll need for your weight workout. Clearly, this is not a very good use of your time in the gym.

I hope you won the bet, I mean... debate. I better get my cut, or I'll have to charge you 3 points vig a week, until you pay up.

Does running on an empty stomach burn more fat?

Question: I recently read an article from one of those "trainer-to-the-stars" guys who said he makes his clients run on an empty stomach to burn more fat. Does that work? I'm not planning to starve myself before workouts, but should I cut out my (healthy) pre-workout snacks to burn more fat at the gym?
Thanks.

~ Angie

Answer: I know some idiot personal trainers are going to be writing in telling me the total opposite because they read it in some stupid magazine. Because everything in those magazines is true, right? But no Virginia, there is no Santa Claus... oops, I think I had too much egg nog, wrong question. The trainer to the stars is himself an idiot. There is no way that the body will burn more fat on an empty stomach and who wants to work out on an empty stomach? You just feel ten times more hungry after the workout.

Exercising on an empty stomach has never been that good for you. Research studies have indicated that the number of calories burned is far less than when exercising after a meal. A small meal of 300-400 calories an hour or so before training will allow you to train harder. You will get about a 10% increase in metabolic rate alone from eating the food, you will be able to train harder as blood glucose levels will not drop like a rock, and you will have a better anabolic hormone response.

Exercising on an empty stomach does not force the body to burn more fat. In some cases it actually forces it to break down more muscle to get at amino acids, which are converted into glucose and then help supply the body with energy. Small amounts of glucose are needed to burn fat (supplying muscle to help move the body).

This has been the technical part of the programming. Now for the layman's part... Do not starve your body when working out and don't listen to those "trainers to the stars," unless of course it's me training those stars.

Most fitness advice is full of crap!

Question: Help! I have heard so much "advice" from people since I started working out again. I have heard you need to: 1.) Work out first thing, before you eat breakfast 2.) Work out anytime in the morning 3.) If you work out before breakfast, you will eat more during the day. 4.) Muscle weighs the same as fat, therefore if you are working out and don't see a change in the scale you need to cut back on calories.

Can you help me clarify these conflicting statements?

~ *Kim*

Answer: Most people that give advice, especially fitness advice, are full of crap. Yes, I will be more than happy to clarify this stupidity. There is no difference if you work out in the morning, afternoon or night. Whenever you feel comfortable and are able to get a good workout is when you should work out. You don't burn more calories because you work out on an empty stomach. Actually I think it's stupid. I like to work out one hour after I've eaten, but that's my preference. You need to do what will give you the best feeling when you're working out.

There are no actual studies that claim that people eat more if they work out before breakfast. I will tell you if you're starving after your workout, eat breakfast the minute you wake up; you'll have more energy for your workout and you won't be starving through the day.

Muscle does not weigh the same as fat; it actually weighs more, almost twice as much per square inch. Whoever told you to cut back on calories is an idiot and should be slapped upside their head. The scale means absolutely nothing when you begin to work out; losing body fat is what counts. Get your body fat checked or take a photo of yourself and compare it every six weeks to the person in the mirror. This will help you chart your progress.

Throw that damn scale away or better yet give it to the idiot that told you that muscle weighs the same as fat. Hopefully you can educate the stupid "advice" giver to the real world. Thanks for playing "You've been given stupid advice"!

Hey, Johnny what does she win for playing? That's right a healthier lifestyle! Congratulations.

He says he's giving me a good workout...

Question: I go to the gym 3 times a week, I have a trainer and he says he is giving me a good workout. I use a lot of machines and I bike... I have only lost 1/2 lb... I want to lose more weight. I have lost 5 inches total. What to do... more cardio? What?

~ Karen

Answer: Many trainers out there are making good money by telling what you *"want"* to hear, not what you *"need"* to hear. One thing you have to know is that your trainer has to tell you he's giving you a good workout. He wants you to keep forking over the money you pay him. In all honesty, I can't assess the situation without more information. Such as, how long have you been going and where was the 5 inches lost? Two things I want you to do. 1.) Ask yourself, do you think he's giving you a good workout and 2.) Tell his stupid ass to start you on some Interval Aerobic Training. If it's on the bike pedal 95 rpm for 2 minutes and then 120 rpm's for 2 minutes and so on until you hit 20 minutes.

From what it reads like, your intensity isn't up to snuff. What does your trainer do, stand there and watch you while counting reps like "Rainman" 1... 2... 3... yea 3, definitely 3. Tell him to drop his clipboard and stop looking at himself in the mirror and maybe *spot* you for a couple of reps or find a trainer that wants to work you hard.

Save your money and don't buy "Animal Cuts"

Question: My 18-year-old son has friends who are taking Animal Cuts. They swear that it works. My son is in great shape; he'd like to be more "cut and defined," he says. What do you know about this product? He thinks it will work, and there are no side effects or steroids. I say just change his workout.
Thanks,
~ *Sue*

Answer: This is a common question asked of me from concerned parents. Every bodybuilder in Cincinnati will be writing nasty letters to me but who gives a shit. I try very hard to not know that much about what goes on in the crazy cultive world of bodybuilding. You have supplement companies selling pipe dreams in glossy ads with professional bodybuilders who take steroids, growth hormones and the like; endorsing and telling 16-year-olds who want to get bigger, stronger and faster that this is the way to paradise. When I was 18 I had more testosterone than I knew what to do with and I was ripped to shreds. Here's a little secret I'll share with you. I lifted hard and consistent, did aerobic training (I ran, even though I hate running) and watched what I put in my mouth (I didn't eat much saturated fat, lots of olive oil, I'm Italian if you didn't suspect) and I made sure I drank plenty of water. When I wanted to bulk up I just ate more food anywhere between 4000 to 8000 calories a day. That's right eat, work out, go to the bathroom about 4-5 times a day. I say add more aerobic activity to his workout and reduce the saturated fat in his diet. Tell him to save his money and have him buy something nice for his girlfriend. If he doesn't have a girlfriend, then make him buy something nice for you. Thank you for being a concerned parent.

My trainer demanded I quit smoking

Question: I went to a local personal trainer recently to try to get help with getting my body in shape. One problem, I smoke. He told me that I needed to stop smoking before he would train me. He said there is no benefit to working out if I didn't stop smoking.
~ *Cheryl*

Answer: Tell the idiot workout Nazi to put away his self-righteousness! If you're willing to commit to an exercise program, I would rather you exercise and smoke than smoke and not exercise. Begin an exercise program and as you continue you will notice that smoking interrupts the positive quality of life changes you're trying to develop. You will feel better when you don't smoke. I will never and don't condone smoking but it is a hard habit to break especially if you have smoked a long time, so go to a trainer that will help you create an exercise program even though you smoke. After the exercise thing has become part of your lifestyle then try a smoking cessation program. Don't be too puritanical in your thinking; it usually leads to failure.

Stretching before cardio?

Question: I've read conflicting reports on if it's appropriate to stretch before a cardio workout. Some say stretching beforehand may help prevent injury during the workout, but others claim that stretching before a cardio session can negatively impact your ability to maintain a higher-intensity workout. Which is true?

~ Angela

Answer: Don't you have other things to worry about? To stress about stretching is not a good use of your time. But because I'm a nice guy I'll answer your question and make the conflict disappear. Stretching usually doesn't need to be done if you warm up and get the blood going. I'm not a big fan of stretching because if you perform a repetition throughout the full range of movement in regards to a specific joint you're creating strength throughout the full range of motion. Increased flexibility comes with getting that muscle stronger to be able to handle more stress that may be placed on it.

There'll be a million idiots out there that will freak out because I've said this and they're still stretching and wasting their time for 30 minutes to go on a 20-minute run. There is such a thing as over-stretching also. But to answer your second question, I haven't seen much evidence to claim that stretching will negatively impact the intensity of your workout. Now go warm up, work out and look HOT for the summer!

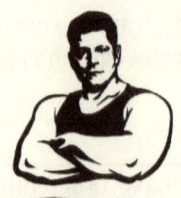

Can You Believe They Asked Me This?

Exercises to re-center my headlights?

Question: Help me out here Roc. I am your average ex-football player kinda guy. Consistently in the home gym doing some sort of weights or cardio virtually everyday. I am 6'2" and 255. I know, I know, not the 185 recommended by the BMI but I am very comfortable in my size... except, my chest. I have a chest that tends to point outwards; my headlights shine against the curb. Is there some sort of exercise I am missing here? I do push-ups, chin-ups, jumping jacks, bench, curls and butterfly presses to work my upper body and chest. I am starting to get the feeling that I am doing some sort of strength training that is promoting my inner chest and not my outer chest... if such a thing exists. Can you advise me on exercises to re-center the headlights here? Should I lay off a particular exercise and work in another? Thanks for the entertaining/knowledgeable advice.

~ *Allen*

Answer: This has to be the craziest friggin' question I've ever gotten. First of all screw the BMI. As long as you feel good at the weight you're at, don't worry. I used to be 225 at 5'9" and felt great. I decided to cut down to 205 for television; you know the whole TV adds 10 pounds crap. The second part of the question disturbs me but I'll answer it anyway. I haven't seen any photos so this is just a guess, but it seems that you've done too much chest and not enough back and shoulders. I would lay off doing too many chest exercises limit your sets to flat bench flyes, 2 sets of 20 and perform lateral raises and rear delt raises. Front Lat (Lattisimus) pulldowns or Horizontal rows. I think your posture is off and if your shoulders come forward it will tend to make the chest look more separated and give that turned headlight look. I hope the hell I did some good here, report back to me in 8 weeks, you should start to see a difference by then.

Should I stop having sex to gain weight?

Question: I have been hitting the gym 3-5 times a week. I have been eating good plus whey twice a day. I am gaining, but would I gain faster if I stopped having sex or should I have more sex?

~ Ben

Answer: O.K idiot boy. Questions like this deserve a huge, and I mean huge slap upside your head. I don't care how fast you want to gain weight you don't stop having sex to achieve it. If you can have more sex then have more sex and make sure it's good sex. Don't just have sex for the fuck of it. No pun intended. Perfect practice makes perfect. Get to the gym and get into bed and have fun doing both. I really don't think the 25 kcals expended during a round of sex is inhibiting your weight gain.

Is my "Unit" in trouble? Boxers or Briefs?

Question: I am 29, I work out regularly and have since high school. I run 12-15 miles a week, bike about 20 miles a week and lift 2 days a week. I was at my gym the other day and while changing in the locker room one of the gym trainers saw that I wear boxer shorts. It appears that he has an issue with boxers; he said that I need to wear something with more support. He claims that I could damage my unit and make it difficult to have children. My girlfriend works out at the same place and he told her. She bought me some briefs. Briefs suck. I went online and have not been able to verify what this trainer told me. Is he full of shit or should I be concerned about my unit? And if so what do you recommend for support?
Thanks
~ *J.C.*

Answer: First of all what the hell is a trainer at your gym doing looking at you in the locker room and why is your "unit" any of his concern? And then to go tell your girlfriend his stupid ass opinion on the boxers vs. briefs controversy, give me a friggin' break. I think he's trying to bang your girlfriend... just sayin'. It depends on what makes you feel comfortable and what activity you are doing. If you're strength training, boxers are fine. I personally enjoy a little more support when I bike and run. I get that support when wearing bike shorts. As long as you don't feel discomfort and your "unit" isn't jostling around and causing you pain I wouldn't worry about it too much. I know I'm going to date myself here but what the hell, here it goes; In that great decade we call the eighties there was a huge controversy about how men's bikini briefs compacted the "unit" and didn't allow it to breath properly and would cause the little swimmers to not be so active. I think that's why Calvin Klein came out with the boxer briefs in 1990. I recommend you do what's comfortable for you and tell the trainer to stop talking to your girlfriend about your "unit." I think there's something a little shady about that either he's trying to get with you or get with your girlfriend.

Exercising your triceps can be a real "turn on."

Question: This is bizarre: whenever I am doing standing triceps kickbacks I get really, really ...umm... turned on-- like I'm also working out my PC muscles. (It's almost too much to bear.) Is there anything to this?
~ Jewel

Answer: I don't think it is bizarre; when you've been in this business as long as I have nothing seems bizarre anymore. Most of the time bizarre to most people is passé in my book. As I have discovered your "turned on" feeling isn't yours alone, many women have complained or bragged about a certain exercise that can get them excited in the gym. Your PC or pubococcygeal muscles (also known as the "pelvic floor") are muscles that, when strengthened or used in a rhythmic clenching and unclenching (called "Kegals" pronounced "ka-gills" named for a Dr. Kegal), can produce a "turned on" effect because (according to experts) these exercises when done correctly produce better, longer and more controlled orgasms. What I can gather is that when you're bent over while performing tricep kick backs your pelvic muscles are used to stabilize your body and with each repetition produces a rhythm in your PC muscles and causes you to get "turned on." I hope it doesn't inhibit your workout; if it does, try something that keeps your body aligned straight up and down, standing or lying down--perhaps a tricep pushdown, or lying tricep press. This is what I can come up with for your little but not so bad of a problem. I have to tell you I've never felt more like Dr. Ruth than right now.

I dealt with being raped at 14

Question: I dealt with being raped at 14 by trying to buff up and joining the weight-lifting classes at my high school. I was informed that being a girl meant I couldn't really build muscle. I was told to go with low weight and high reps, but I figured if I was going to bother I should go with high weight. After 3 years I felt confident enough about me to shed the baggy men's clothing that had helped me feel safe in favor of a more feminine look. But I had gained muscle, think She-man in a spaghetti-strap dress. I tried to make it work anyway despite the total strangers who were amused by, or abusive about "that cross dresser". But after being detained by cops because I matched the description of the "young man" who had just robbed the gas station, my self-esteem was shot. I graduated 3 years ago, and have since gained 50 pounds. Now I want to lose it, but what I really want is to lose the muscle mass. Is there any way to do that without damaging my heart? Is there any way to safely lose fat and muscle together? Or should I just lose the weight and start wearing leather 24/7?
~ *Elise*

Answer: I'm not sure where to start! I'm really bummed out about the rape and would love to make whoever that was a bloody spot on the pavement. Then I'd like to slap the crap out of strangers for being so stupid. Last but not least I'd give anything to pee in the cop's coffee that couldn't see that you were a young lady. O.K., now that I set the record straight and have made three new enemies let's get on to answering the question: Keep the muscle lose the fat. I doubt very much that you looked like a she-man. Lucy Lawless as Xenia: Warrior Princess, two words... HOT and Hot. If you haven't noticed there are many more fat people than that appear to be any in some kind of shape. So I wouldn't put too much credence into fat people commenting on how fit people look.

Yes... to the question about doing something without damaging your heart but I would not want to lose the muscle. Muscle is the greatest fat burner we have. Yes there are ways to lose fat and muscle together. Just go on any ridiculous calorie-restricting diet and don't exercise. That's sure to do wonders for your look. Stay with a program that you can live with and eat sensibly; gaining fifty pounds doesn't come from eating sensibly. About the leather, keep it for when you're feeling a tad bit sassy.

Will people burn more fat if they strength train first?

Question: Hi Rocco: I have a question about your column from a week ago. You said that people should always do the strength workout first, and by doing so more fat will be burned during the cardio workout.

Will people really burn more fat during the cardio workout if they lift first? If someone has a good high-carbo diet, won't there be enough glycogen left in the muscles and the liver for both workouts?

Which leads me to the next question: Why does it matter if someone burns a fat calorie or a carbo calorie, as long as the total number of calories spent is the same? If one day I run 10 sprints and burn 100kcals - all from glycogen, then walk a mile at 3 ½ mph the next day and burn 100 kcals - from carbos and fat, what difference does it make? I burned the same number of calories.

I have one final question, and I'd appreciate an answer, because I always hear different explanations for this: If someone is in good aerobic condition and he/she jogs at a moderate intensity, will all the cals in the first 15-17 mins be from carbs? It doesn't make sense that it would take the same amount of time for everyone. If someone is in good shape and jogs at an easy pace, won't fat be used as a fuel within a few minutes - along with carbs?

I apologize for the long-winded email, but I'd appreciate your feedback. I want to make sure I'm doing the right things and giving other people the right info. Thanks,
~ *Dave*

Answer: You have got to be kidding me! Not all calories are the same. What rock did you crawl out from under? It depends on what your needs are for energy. If you're fat you probably would want to burn more fat than glycogen. If staying with your stupid theory that all calories were the same, then burning protein calories would be a good thing. And it isn't. I'm really not sure which question to answer first because they're all kind of goofy but I'll give it my best shot.

1) Yes. People will burn more fat if they lift first; I would not have wrote that if it weren't true. Most people waste so much time doing aerobics first.

2) Yes. Your body should have enough glycogen stores for both workouts but it has more to do with efficiency (less time in the gym) and burning more fat in a shorter amount of time.

3) Depending on the fitness of the person it may take a shorter amount of time to begin utilizing fat during a sustained aerobic workout. The 13-17 minutes is just a gauge; not everyone is the same, especially unfit people.

Any other questions I can answer for you? There's probably one you left out.

I'm a skinny piece of shit. How do I gain weight?

Question: First of all, I would like to ask you what my best bet would be to gain some weight. I know this may be an odd question, but realistically, I'm a skinny piece of shit. I am 5'9 and my weight varies between 135 to 150, and no matter what I do, I don't gain any weight. I even have tried lifting weights and exercising, but my metabolism is extremely high. Is there anything I can do to put on some weight, the healthy kind, of course? My goal is to be about 170 or 180 of pure muscle or close to it. As is right now, I am scrawny, but still muscular for my size. What should I do?

~ *Mike*

Answer: Hey Mike, I'm the only one that can use profanity here. To get to your question and to let you in on a little secret, skinny pieces of shit are called "Hardgainers" in my business. And the only way that "Hardgainers" can gain muscle weight is by eating as many calories as you can consume and keeping the workout very simple. Train two exercises per body part with high intensity. Eat tons of carbs because they are considered protein sparing, which will help you to gain more muscle. Too many idiots suck down too much protein because they think that will help them gain more muscle, in a word...STUPID! LIFT HARD: EAT MORE that's pretty much the formula for you Mike. Get going and keep me posted.

My husband loves my "Assets." How do I get him to back off?

Question: I've always been good looking, but I've been working out 3x a week and eating much better than I ever have. I'm 5'8" and 136 lbs. My husband of 11 years has always nicely complimented me on my "assets," but now he is constantly hounding me. I don't have time for this as I have two kids, a job and a house to take care of. Should I slow down on the working out or how else can I get him to back off?

~ Marcy

Answer: This is a tough one, Marcy. Most women I talk to are always complaining that they can't get their husbands to pay any attention to them let alone hound them. After 11 years that's pretty good. I'm no marriage counselor but not working out is definitely not the answer. Keep working out and looking great but I think you should sit down with your husband and figure out a schedule that is suitable for the both of you. I've seen women try to gain weight and the husband decides to go looking elsewhere. Just like working out there needs to be time for "it." I don't mind hearing a little tinge of selfishness on your part, a marriage is a give and take and sometimes compromises have to be made. But by no means is stopping working out a solution. Your workout is for "you" and no one else. And how else are you going to keep up with those two kids?

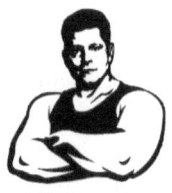

Dumbbells... and Treadmills... and Rubber Bands... Oh My!

Just give me the Algebra, I'll do the math myself

Question: I have recently started riding a stationary bike and ski machine every day 20 minutes each, and I have a whole bunch of questions for you.

> 1. I am wondering how to track/estimate the calories I burn? Everything I find concerning the bike asks mph but my bike only tells rpm. Could you tell me how to convert rpm to mph. My best guess is 1mile/circumfrence (of wheel)x60=MPH but I have never been good at algebra so I don't know.
>
> 2. Does a ski machine count as down hill, cross-country, or Nordic? I know that's a dumb question but I have never had any interest in skiing and don't know the *#%@* difference.
>
> 3. There is all this Watt NM KJ stuff on my bike. I know it has something to do with energy consumption, but what?
>
> 4. I am considering a career in dietetics (although I do have a lot to learn) do they make good money?

Also it may help you to know that my skier is a stamina 885 and my bike a Tunturi, and on the bike I try to keep my settings at 60RPM 20-25NM & 100-150 Watt. If you could just give me the algebraic expression I'll do the math myself. I greatly appreciate your help and your work, and I apologize for all the questions, I just don't know who else to ask. Thanks.

~ Katie

Answer: Holy Crap! My friggin' head is spinning! I sucked at Algebra; it took me twice to get through the damn class. It didn't help that I was in a juvenile detention center for half of the first year of it. But I know I still hate Algebra. I can give you the estimate depending on your weight but I see you conveniently left that out, so you are SOL on that question. Next: Ski machines are supposedly simulating cross-country-style skiing. The term MET is short for Metabolic equivalent; an MET is a unit of energy or level of oxygen used at rest (1 MET = VO_2 of 3.5 mL/kg/min). Watts is the amount of work you are doing or the workload you have placed on yourself. Dietitians and Nutritionists make good money and we need as many as we can get so keep studying. You need to ramp your RPM's up to at least 90 RPM's unless you're on death's door. I would also recommend using a heart rate monitor instead of trying to do all this crazy math. You can buy one very inexpensively at your local fitness store. It just makes it easier to track and gauge your progress.

What is an E-Z Bar French Press?

Question: What is an E-Z Bar French press? What is a close-grip bench push-up?
~ *Kevin*

Answer: You know that's two questions, and on The Burbank Show I would have blown you up, but since I'm trying to be a nice guy, I'll answer them both. An E-Z Bar French Press has something lewd to do with a bistro, sluts, newspaper editors and I think midgets but that's way out of my league. I don't know why you'd be asking me that question, you must be sick! Oh, oh, the exercise equipment, yeah, that's easy. An E-Z bar is a curling bar that has two indents in the middle of the bar that look like triangles. This bar was invented to make curling more comfortable and help isolate the bicep muscle. The French press is a tricep exercise that is usually done with a dumbbell (and not your little brother) placing both arms straight over your head and bending at the elbow so that the dumbbell is behind your head and just barely misses giving you a concussion on every rep. So now that you know that.

An E-Z Curl French Press would be performed by placing your hands on the inside part of the triangle indents and gripping the bar and trying to bend at the elbows balancing a bar and not separating your shoulder and giving yourself a concussion. Good luck! I'm not sure which close-grip bench push-up exercise this goofball is telling you to do so I'll give you the one I think he is, since I have my crystal ball sitting next to me. There are four that I know of. But I digress. A close-grip bench push-up is performed by placing your hands on the side of a bench about two inches apart, face toward the bench (looking down) keeping your legs straight and bending at the elbows. Make sure that your chest is over your hands. If your head is over your hands you're sure to get a broken nose when your triceps fatigue. So don't do that. I'm glad to be of service.

When using Nautilus machines...

Question: I have increased my weight-training sessions, which last about 30 minutes, to 3 times a week. When using Nautilus machines, should I do one rep with heavy weight until the point of exhaustion (about 8-10 lifts) or 2-3 reps with tolerable weights? My goal is to tone my muscles and increase my strength.

~ *TJ*.

Answer: It's obvious to me that you haven't been in the exercise game long or you would know the difference between a rep and a set. I won't break your chops too much because at least you're doing something, not like the 80% of humans on this planet that sit on their ass and eat fast food.

There is a little education needed here for the new people getting into exercise. Repetitions are the actual performance of an exercise and when you group these repetitions together, they are considered a set. With the lesson out of the way here's the answer to your question. There's been a raging debate over this exact question since the 1970's when Arthur Jones, the founder and inventor of Nautilus, started promoting his product. I'm a fan of the one set to exhaustion but there is nothing bad to say about multiple set training except that it wastes a lot of time. If you like being in the gym, do multiple sets; if you want to get pretty much the same results and get out of the gym in half the time, do the higher intensity workout. Either one will get you to your goal, it just depends on how hard to you want to work.

Use what you got and forget the gym memberships.

Question: My wife and I are expecting our first child in October, and in a cost-cutting move, we've both cancelled our gym memberships. Now, we have some equipment at home (a weight bench, a treadmill, and Gazelle-type machine), and we're looking to use it more. Is it possible to get a solid workout with these pieces?

We're used to visiting the gym 4-5 times a week with a routine on the machines. How do we translate that workout to our home equipment? Any help is much appreciated.

~ Anthony

Answer: If you had all this equipment in the first place why didn't you use it sooner? Instead you wasted your money on the equipment in the first place and then wasted money on gym memberships. It's funny, when life-changing situations happen (like having a baby) we get back to basics. Getting back to basics is where we should be in the first place. If you add some dumbbells to what you already have you can definitely get a solid workout. I would suggest you call a qualified fitness professional to help you with the workout. You haven't given me real specifics of the equipment so I'm a little hesitant to give a full-blown workout. One question though, how the hell did you get sucked into buying a Gazelle? I guess that new credit card was burning a hole in your pocket or just drinking at three in the morning with nothing better to do. To answer your question about translating the workout from the gym to the home equipment, you don't. You create a new one utilizing the equipment you have available.   Good luck with the workout and the new baby. I hope the baby is healthy and learns to use that equipment with you.

What you're doing on the treadmill is called "Interval Training."

Question: I'm trying to lose 25 lbs and I have been doing weight/strength training. I hate cardio but have started to force myself to do at least 40 minutes of boring treadmill. I start by walking 5 minutes then run for 3 then walk for 2 then run 3... you get it. This wears me out! Way more than regular running. Is this a good way to lose my weight? Should I incorporate something else? Also I try to eat well and add a protein shake in the mix from time to time.

~ **Nikki,** *Phoenix, Arizona*

Answer: Nikki... what the hell are you doing writing me from Phoenix, Arizona? Aren't there any trainers there that you can ask this question to? Obviously the 120-degree heat must be getting to them because this is a pretty easy question to answer. What you're doing on the treadmill is called interval training and it is probably the best way to trick your body into losing fat. When you stay on a treadmill or the street for a sustained period of time, your body will get used to that and will not burn as much fat as you continue your training. When you include interval training as part of your regiment, your body is thrown into chaos and has no idea what to do, so it burns fat. You don't need to run more than 20 – 25 minutes doing interval training because it does kick your ass. One tip I'd like to give you is get off the treadmill sometimes and go to a bike or elliptical trainer to add some variety to the boring aerobic workout. I hate aerobic training also, but if you need to lose fat you need to do it. Most importantly, be consistent and don't give up and you will see amazing results. Do me a favor and tell someone to put the air conditioning on in Phoenix. I hate any place that I can cook my breakfast on the pavement.

What's the difference between "Fat Burning" and "Aerobic"?

Question: The equipment I use at the gym (Arc; EFX; treadmill) offers various user programs, including "aerobic" and "fat burning." What's the difference? Thanks.

~ Mark

Answer: You, as well as most of us in the fitness industry, don't exactly know what the equipment manufacturers are talking about. It's funny because you'll see in an advertisement that a treadmill has two "fat burning" and two "aerobic" programs. I can see if there's scenery and they're taking you through the south of France or maybe Tuscany. I don't even know if people use the programs any more. In my training programs I usually use the manual program and create my own. Here's the best answer that I could come up with. Supposedly, the equipment manufacturers create the "Fat Burning" to help a 150-lb individual to work at 50-60% of his maximum heat rate where the body primarily uses fat stores for energy. This is supposed to produce more fat burning with less fatigue. The "aerobic" program takes your heart rate between 65-85% of maximum heart rate where the body shifts to using stored glycogen and less fat and the workout on the heart and lungs are pushed to their beneficial limits. Obviously this is there to increase your aerobic fitness. Is this true? It's hard to say because all the programs are set for an average 150-lb person. Depending on your fitness level, weight and amount of muscle you're carrying around, fat burning may actually be an "aerobic" workout for you. I recommend you see a qualified fitness professional and first figure out what type of shape you're in, instead of leaving it up to a treadmill.

What is the best Elliptical Trainer for the buck?

Question: Since it is a new year, fitness is always the big thing this time of year. What do you feel is the best Home Elliptical Trainer for the buck? I really don't want to spend over $500-$700. Thanks.
~ Brad

Answer: Ahhhh... The New Year and the floodgates open with questions about what to buy and how to get fit on the cheap. It's obvious to me that you're new to my column, an askROCCO virgin so to speak. Because if you weren't you would have read at least six of my columns that pertain to starting an exercise program first, staying committed to that program, seeing results and then maybe purchasing some sort of fitness equipment that floats your fancy. For the record, I recommend that you do NOT buy an elliptical trainer at this time. Instead, go to my RoccoCastellano.com blog, look through the archived articles and find a workout that agrees with you.

However, if you really are hell-bent on purchasing an elliptical trainer, do yourself a favor and save up your money and buy a real one. $500-$700 dollars will buy you nothing more than a pile of plastic and metal. The saying, "you get what you pay for" really rings true when buying fitness equipment. After two years, at the very best you will have a broken trainer and at the very least a ridiculously expensive clothes rack. I'm going to give you a little math lesson for the new year, so hold on to those No. 2 pencils.

Let's say you purchase an elliptical trainer from some big sporting goods store (which shall remain nameless) for $500 dollars. In pricing that piece of equipment, the store has done something called key stoning. This means that they bought the trainer for only $250 and then doubled its cost for their consumer. They're a retailer, that's what they do. Usually, manufacturers will double the cost minus 45 percent. This is what it looks like in simple mathematical terms: 250 divided by 2 = 125 – 45% = 81. $81! You just paid $500 for an elliptical trainer that cost the manufacturer only $81 to make. Unfortunately, I can guarantee that you'll be buying another $500 ($81) elliptical trainer in two years.

If you are serious about exercise, invest more money and buy one that will last for a long time. On the other hand, if you're not so serious about exercise, save your money, go shopping and buy some new outfits, because you'll get much more use out of them.

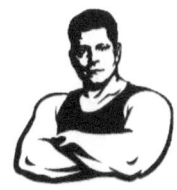

I'm No Doctor and
I Don't Play One on T.V.
(and exercising before and after injury)

Good thing for my trusty crystal ball

Question: I'm 37 and weigh 156. I want to tone up and strengthen my muscles but I have a bad back and don't know what kind of exercises I can do that would help me. I walk every day but that isn't enough. If you could give me some exercises I would be so thrilled. I am starting Yoga on Monday.

~ Teresa

Answer: I believe I made reference to the phrase "tone up," "toning up" or anything related to those words in previous columns but I'll give you a refresher course. Once again, for the reading impaired, those words were some marketing genius' way of making strength training or muscle building more palatable for you women folk. It's an annoying phrase because I think all women should strength train to shape their muscles and the only way to do that is by building muscle. Now on to the actual meat of the question. You haven't provided me with any specifics about your bad back, so I'll look into my crystal ball and try to figure out what part of your back is bad. Ahhhh! There it is! Your lower lumbar, (good thing I had my trusty crystal ball). There are two specific exercises that I recommend that can be done anywhere.

1. **The Swimmer:** Lie face down on a mat or the floor (if you don't like sucking on rug fibers place your forehead on a small pillow). With your arms above your head and legs slightly apart (your body should resemble an "X") raise your right arm and left leg simultaneously keeping your head on the pillow or

face sucking fibers, repeat this for 20 repetitions. When you have completed 20 reps, switch and raise your left arm and right leg. Now isn't this fun for the whole family!

2. **Superman:** Stay lying face down sucking rug fibers, and raise both hands and both legs at the same time very slowly (keep your legs and arms as straight as possible); do not make any jerking movements or the exercise police will come to your house and smack you upside the head. Perform this exercise for 20 repetitions also. When your back is starting to feel stronger write me back so I can give you the rest of your strength-training workout. Coupled with a strength workout, walking at various speeds will be enough aerobic activity.

My self-diagnosis is "Fatigue Disease"

Question: I have a serious lack of energy these days, even though I typically get 7-8 hours of sleep, eat very healthy (no junk food) and work out 3-5 days per week...strength training and cardio. My self-diagnosis is this "fatigue disease" could be attributed to the fact that I stare at a computer for 8 hours a day. My eyes are numb! How do you find that extra energy to aid you for night workouts or going out?

~ Kate

Answer: This problem is nothing new. Many people feel beat up after working an environment that is not conducive to what their body wants. Most bodies need to do physical work with their energy needs being met. If it is possible I would recommend you try to get your workouts done in the morning or at lunchtime and eat small meals throughout the day. Stay away from caffeine and sugar, as these chemicals tend to sap your energy by the end of the day. As a side note: Try taking a walk every two hours during your work day, get some blood moving and you won't feel so sluggish. If your boss complains, tell him or her that smokers get ten-minute breaks every five minutes, and you being a "non-smoker" want to take some time to try and stay healthy. If they can suck on cancer sticks to relieve their stress then you can take a walk. If you can't take a walk try to do 50 to 100 jumping jacks; this should definitely get your blood pumping.

Should I follow my Doctor's advice?

Question: Rocco, I'm a recently divorced woman whose kids have all left or are at college. For years, I was focused on my kids or my husband -- making sure dinner was on the table and the kids' schoolwork was done or they were on time for soccer, band, football or whatever. I let myself come last. Now that it's just me I've had to be honest and take stock of my lifestyle. I'm about 30 pounds overweight and the curves are in all the wrong places. My doctor tells me to start walking or trying aerobics. But, you say people who are overweight shouldn't walk because it's bad for their knees. Should I follow my DR's advice or ignore it? And do aerobics put pressure on my knees? And what do you think of Pilates or yoga? Thanks.

~ Connie

Answer: Those damn husbands… you cook, you clean and who knows what the hell else. Well Connie, it's about time you focus on you and let's not focus on walking (or at least for the time being). You are correct in stating that I'm not a big fan of people that are overweight just jumping into a walking program. Walking places undue stress on you lower back, hips, knees and ankles. What I suggest you do is work on strengthening or building muscle in those areas before beginning a walking program. While you're strengthening your muscles to absorb the shock of the pounding from walking you should ride a bicycle or elliptical trainer for an aerobic activity. If these are not available to you, do the strength-training program first, build the muscle and then begin your walking program. My opinion on Pilates and yoga is to have at it. These can be part of the muscle strengthening that I advised. In this case I would ignore your doctor's advice.

Weight gain after Gastric Bypass

Question: 18 months ago I had gastric bypass surgery. I was over 360 lbs and I am now down to my goal of 190. Now I want to put on some weight. I've been going to my local gym 3-4 days a week since May. I've noticed I've gotten stronger, but I can't seem to get bigger. Mainly I want to have defined arms, shoulders, and chest. I've got a pretty good routine where I do 2 body parts per day, 5 different exercises per body part and 4 sets of 8-12 reps on each of those. I think my problem may be protein intake. Due to my eating restrictions, I can't get in much. I drink 3 whey protein shakes a day with skim milk (about 32 grams of protein in each) and eat nothing but chicken and fish for the most part. Please help me!

~ Josh

Answer: Josh, I have to tell you, it sucks. It has nothing to do with your protein intake; it has everything to do with food intake in general. In order for your body to repair muscle that has been broken down from the stress of exercise, you need nutrition or in another word "food." If you don't take in enough you will never build muscle. I hear this so much from gastric bypass patients and I tell them that hindsight is twenty-twenty. If you would have consulted me before the operation I would have told you to go to the gym and build as much muscle as you could because it's so much easier building muscle when you're heavier. Then if you wanted to still get the operation you would have went in with the muscle you needed. I don't know why doctors don't tell you this but it drives me crazy because I'm not against Gastric Bypass surgery if you have exhausted everything in your being to losing the fat. Still though, it still is a calories in, calories expended formula that has been around for thousands of years and will be for thousands more. I probably sound so friggin' preachy right now I think I better tell you how to fix your problem.

You need to eat more carbs not protein! (vegetables, fruits and the like); next you need to be doing more reps. 4 sets of 8-12 is just idiotic, and I know someone that you thought had a brain told you to do this, well STOP! 2 sets of 15-20 will break down the muscle sufficiently and cause muscle hypertrophy (building of muscle). One other note the body needs to work in tandem with itself so going to a full-body workout may prove to be more beneficial. I hope this helps, and you doctors out there: Maybe before you recommend a procedure you may want to talk to fitness professionals.

My skin isn't bouncing back

Question: I had gastric bypass surgery in April and have lost 100 lbs. I still have about 40 to go. However, at the age of 46, I find my skin isn't bouncing back the way I'd hoped. What should I be doing to firm up all this extra skin since plastic surgery isn't a realistic option?

~ Jackie

Answer: Well, Jackie, if you want the skin to bounce back before 18-24 months then plastic surgery better be an option. This is a dilemma for me because I hate plastic surgery; I think it's a wussy way to get rid of fat or to look younger. The problem is there is no way to get rid of extra skin naturally except for time. The body is not made to lose fat quickly no matter what that idiot Dr. Atkins or any other Doctor tells you. Your skin is an organ that grows as you grow in fatness. Getting rid of excess skin is a slow process for the body because it is not a process that the human body was made to do. So if plastic surgery is not an option then my advice is to keep exercising and be patient; it will eventually come back to its natural state.

My knees are making creaking noises...

Question: I am a 40-year-old man who is returning to the gym after a long layoff. I have been using the elliptical trainer for about 30 minutes every day. Now, when I go up and down stairs, my knees are making creaking noises, but I have no knee pain.

I have not been stretching before working out, but I am going to start doing that.

Is there anything else I can do?

~ *Steve*

Answer: First of all, what the hell took you so long getting back to the gym? At 40 I think everyone has something creaking on them. Our bodies are like old doors, maybe still functional but awful noisy when neglected. I'll be 40 years old soon and many things creak on me and I'm in pretty good shape. From what I know about hitting the gym after a long layoff, you need to always strengthen the joints before you hit any aerobic equipment. This will always add more stability to the joint you are trying to protect and avoid the sounds of an aging body. I would avoid stretching the knee joint too much because there's obviously a point of friction that's causing the creaking sounds and you can overstretch the knee joint and cause more damage. When you have the inclination I would check out an orthopedic physician just to make sure there is no degenerative stuff going on.

I think your Doctor would agree

Question: I am scheduled to have knee surgery in mid June, and my doctor and physical therapist have limited me to riding an exercise bike for only ten minutes per day. Besides the other knee exercises they have me doing, can you give me any other exercises to substitute for the running and biking that I used to do? I feel I am putting on some bad weight without my normal cardio routine.

~ *Tyler*

Answer: What the hell is wrong with you? Your doctor and physical therapist both tell you not to do something and then you write and ask me to go against them and give you exercises. It was probably the running that got you here in the first place, and runners drive me crazy. They'll over-train, get injured and then want someone to fix their problems. Arghhhh! I'm not going to give you any exercises because you don't need them, right now. Your real problem is you exercised so much that you needed to take in so many calories to keep your body able to train. Well know your brain and body is still taking in those calories and you don't realize it. Here's my advice, get a food journal (you can get one free by going to RoccoCastellano.com) and write down what you eat. You'll then realize you're taking in way too many calories and upon that realization cut your caloric intake by about 200 calories for the first week and then another 200 the next week. You should be able to maintain your weight for a while until you are fully rehabbed and can start cycling again. (Did you notice I said cycling and not running? I think your doctor would agree.) Good Luck.

Bad back... Blood thinners... what else?

Question: My husband injured his back about 5 years ago. Now he cannot walk but a short distance and cannot stand for any length of time. He has gained considerable amount of weight during this time. He is 6ft. and weighs approximately 340 lbs. and is 59 years old. He also has an irregular heartbeat and is on blood thinners. He wants to lose the weight but does not know what to do. We have tried to eat differently but without exercise it is not helping. Please tell me how to help him because I don't want to lose him to this weight problem. He has a lot of trouble breathing also.

~ Elise

Answer: This is a real bummer, because I don't think that I can help either. I do have several ideas but they're only suggestions and remember that I am not a doctor and will never pretend to be.

- One thing to remember is if you are not expending calories you do not need to take in that many. Your best bet would be to go to a licensed dietician and get the correct caloric intake for him.
- Second, if he can only walk a short distance, keep him walking, let him walk until he can't, let him sit and rest, then get his ass up again. Every day push a little harder, nothing too crazy just a little more each day. It will feel like an eternity but I'll bet within six months he'll be walking easier and feeling better.

The fat won't come off that fast but you need to get to the starting line if you want to finish the race. Let's get your man to the starting line and then we'll figure out how to run the race. This is his journey, stay by his side because he will need a little help along the way. Keep me updated.

Runners and heavy objects don't mix

Question: I'm a regular runner and in good shape. Recently I was lifting boxes and strained my lower back. How can I strengthen my back without going to a gym or buying a fancy weight machine? Are there exercises I can do with small hand weights at home to strengthen my back? (And please don't give me the lecture about the rules of lifting properly or I'll feel the need to give you the lecture about preaching to your readers. Thank you.)

~ Marci

Answer: First of all who the hell do you think you are dictating what I can lecture and what I can't? I know you think you're a feisty little breed of a woman but take a chill pill because I really don't care how people lift heavy objects because no one listens any way. If they did, chiropractors would be out of business. Now getting back to your real question, what can you do to fix your back, am I right? It is my opinion that because you are a runner you probably have tight hamstrings and buttocks. I say this because most runners do not strength train because they believe running is the only way to really stay in shape. Most often then not running actually causes more problems than it needs to but we can't forget that "runner's high," now can we? There's something going on here that you are probably completely unaware of. It's called the domino effect. In a nutshell, it's one body part causing another body part to be in pain or cause discomfort. If your hamstrings are tight (which they probably are!) your hips will become tight and then your lower back becomes tight and before you know it, the stress you place on a tight back (like lifting heavy things) causes you to injure your back. My recommendation to you right now is to let your back rest. Perform exercises that work the hamstrings throughout their full range of motion or stretching your hamstrings while lying on your back (do not reach and bend down towards your knee because you'd be putting more strain on the back you just injured). Lay back and pull on your heel towards your head with a towel, rope or anything that will hold your heel. The more flexible your hamstrings and hips are, the less stress you place on your back. So keep lifting heavy objects because you'll give me more content for columns to come.

I don't want to die at an early age...

Question: I need help. I am a 41-year-old man diagnosed with diabetes. I have been struggling with my weight loss for sometime. Back in November I joined a fitness center with my niece. For 3 months I was working out 3 to 4 times a week; I even got a personal trainer and started feeing good about me, but the eating habits were still there, and I have only been to the gym once since early March. My doctor says I need to lose about 60-70 lbs. To me I think that is a lot but then again if it helps me to get off my medicines for diabetes and other meds I can do it. This is my question: I need HELP, Serious Help; I do not want to die at an early age like my parents did. Any suggestions, and can you help me? Since askROCCO has come out I have been reading your articles every week, this is where I got the encouragement to write to you.

~ Howard

Answer: First of all, I applaud your efforts so far, but I have to say get your ass back to the gym because consistency is what will take the fat off, not some great workout from Rocco. I can give you all the encouragement in the world and all the greatest workouts but without discipline you will die young. I'm not sure if 60 lbs is the actual fat loss that you need. Let's say for argument's sake it is. I'm going to do a little math here for you (and I know what you're saying: "I read askROCCO for the entertainment not to actually learn something"). Bear with me here. You exercise performing strength-training movements 3 days a week, supplement that with some bike riding two days a week (don't go over 30 minutes each workout) on average you'll lose 1.5 pounds per week (I said average all you crazy people); there's 52 weeks in a year. So 52 multiplied by 1.5 equals 72 pounds. Now let's say you only lost an average of 1 stinking pound per week and here's the hard part of the math; 52 multiplied by 1 leaves 52 pounds lost in one year. That, my friend, is what consistency and discipline bring; 52 pounds of fat gone... arrivederci, bye, bye baby. It took you much longer to put that fat on and in only one year you'll be adding years to your life. Hey Howard, good luck on this journey. Write back, my readers would like to check your progress.

I have a hard time exercising with Hypoglycemia...

Question: Yo Rocco! I have hypoglycemia and have a very hard time exercising. After just a few (10 to 15) minutes, I can feel my sugar dropping. I've tried eating before exercise and that helps some, but not enough. I have also noticed a drop in my energy level through the day. I eat fairly healthy and control my "condition" with diet. I've maintained my weight for several years, but I'd like to lose about 15 pounds. I'm a large framed guy, 6 feet tall and I weigh about 225. Any suggestions? Sorry to be long winded.

~ Rich

Answer: Well, Rich you obviously listen to The Gary Burbank Show on 700WLW. Let me tell you, you're not long winded. You should see some of the novels I get telling me life stories from when someone lost their little doll Daisy when they where one year old to how their ex-spouse left them for a younger model, but I digress. I actually struggled with hypoglycemia for several years when I was younger. I don't want to bore you to tears with the chemical processes that relate to this problem but let me try to offer some relief.

Try not to perform your strength-training exercises all at once; stagger each group of muscles (e.g. chest) in between aerobic activity. Something similar to: Dumbbell bench press, walking uphill for 8 minutes, Horizontal row, 8 minutes on treadmill and so on. Don't perform more than 8-10 exercises for the strength training and you should be fine. Try to keep the exercises as compound movements (movements that include multiple joints while performing them, as do the exercises mentioned above). Try not to drink any sports drinks while working out; they only contribute to fluctuating sugar levels. Keep in touch. Your fellow readers will probably want an update.

What can I do at the gym with a broken foot?

Question: I have a broken foot and will be having surgery in three weeks. I need to have 3 pins put in my foot due to a car accident back in December. I have not been able to work out since the accident. I used to run 5 days a week and lift weights. I am losing muscle and starting to gain weight. I will be on crutches for 2 months. Is there any type of exercise that I can do to keep off the weight and try to gain back some muscle?
~ Annette

Answer: No! Psyche! Of course there things you can do, but I won't tell you. Ha... Ha... No really. I'm just trying to break some chops. What are you going to do -- run after me and slap me upside my head? Come on you have a broken foot. I know, with a friend like me, who needs enemies? Back to the question: You can probably do most exercises on selectorized equipment at the gym. Most important to remember is not to do any weight-bearing exercises that pertain to the foot, such as leg press, lunges, running or walking on the treadmill. If your gym has an upper-body ergometer or rowing machine, you may be able to utilize those apparatus without pain or potential re-injury and still get a pretty good aerobic workout. Don't give up; your condition is only temporary and you'll be back out there kickin' ass in no time.

Coming back from Cardiac surgery

Question: I'm in my 50's -- had bypass surgery over a year ago and have been walking and working out. Mainly some cardio (treadmill, bike, stairclimber) and some weights.

I haven't consulted a trainer, because I'm cheap. However, I am maintaining the basic "package" that cardio rehab had me doing a year ago.

I feel that I should be doing more -- don't know why -- but don't we always feel that way? Total workout is 30 minutes of cardio and about 20 of weights 3 times a week. (Plus some additional walking during my "off" days.) Is this enough or should I be doing more?

I don't care about a better body (I'm 6'3" and about 178 pounds, so that ain't a problem), but I do care about a healthier heart. Any advice?

~ Mark

Answer: Increasing the intensity is a tricky subject when coming back from bypass surgery. Most people begin to feel better and think they can take on the world. Or at least think they can get back to hitting the weights hard. I'm happy to hear that you've been doing the cardio rehab package that was given to you for the past year because now your body is asking you to give it more intensity and wants to get stronger. Like Martha Stewart says when she's not doing time, "that's a good thing." Too many people, especially men (because we can be stupid) will go too hard too fast and wind up screwing everything the doctors just fixed.

Before you do start anything that I'm about to tell you, please, and everyone out there over 45 listen up also because a heart attack can be just around the corner for you too, get another stress test and ask them to provide increased intensities like a "Bruce Protocol" on the treadmill to see where you are. After you're cleared for takeoff you can try this or a variation of this workout. Warm up for about 6 to 8 minutes. When you've broken a sweat, do either lunges (on the same leg) or a horizontal leg press (do not use a hip sled, 45-degree press or squats, these put too much stress on the heart without much benefit). Also perform leg extensions and leg curls with each set -- about 25 repetitions, not more than 2 sets (increase the weight or reps not the sets) and get in some chest exercises like chest flyes and dumbbell chest press for 20 reps 2 sets. Back and shoulder exercises are also something I recommend. I'm not going to give you a whole workout since you where too cheap to hire a personal trainer, but more importantly I want you to do a little research on your own. Make sure that you don't spend more than 30 seconds resting between sets, and I definitely think you're on your way to a stronger, healthier heart.

You have to be F**kin' Kidding me!

Question: I am a 19-year-old male. I'm about 6'2", and have a medium build. My goal is to gain muscle, but be lean enough so that the muscles show. I have been lifting for about 3 months and I have a few questions/problems. I lift Mon., Wed., and Fri. I do push-ups, arm curls, lat pull down, military press, shoulder rolls, bench-press, and butterflys. I do these with medium to heavy weights. I was wondering if this schedule might be overworking certain muscle groups. Should I substitute different ones or just drop some all together? Do you suggest on each workout increasing the weight or reps? On certain lifts I am up to 27 reps; I didn't know if that was too many.

I have been having some problems too. When I first started lifting I would sweat a lot, but now I don't sweat very much. Is that normal? Is it normal to be sort of dizzy after lifting? Also, when I first started I would feel a little sick after working out, but I never did. But my last couple times I get really hot and then got sick. I haven't changed anything. The only thing I could think of was that I was on Christmas break from school and got out of my routine, so there was about 2 weeks without lifting. When I started up again, I picked up where I left off. Can your stamina go down in two weeks? Also I lift in the morning when I get up. Can hunger make you sick? Sorry if I am rambling. I would also like to start running and working out my legs. Would doing both of those on Tues. and Thurs. be overworking things too much? Any suggestions on lifting for the back or anything else to improve my workout? Sorry for the long email. Thanks a lot for any help you can give me.
~ *Brian*

118

Answer: You have to be f**kin' kidding me! I don't think my editor has the column space for me to answer this novel adequately. I think I feel sort of dizzy just trying to understand everything you're asking me. I think I need an aspirin or a bat to hit you over the head with. I'm going to answer this in the order of the paragraphs so not to lose mine and the readers' place. Here goes.

If you're doing push-ups you don't need to do bench press; it's redundant. Anything with the arms should be done after the larger muscle groups (chest, back, shoulders) are exhausted. Where is anything for the tricep? Add a tricep press in the mix there, Sport. Increase the weight about 5% when you can do 20 reps easily. There are two reasons you may not be sweating:

> 1) Your body's not working as hard as it did when you began this exercise program.
>
> 2) You're not drinking enough water throughout the day as well as during the workout (this can also be contributing to you becoming dizzy). Drink at least half your body weight in ounces per day and that should help. If not go see a doctor.

It's not very likely that you lost that much stamina or muscle in two weeks unless you were partying like a Rock Star and didn't sleep for the two weeks you were off. Yes hunger can make you sick if you work out hard. Try to eat a little something when you get up (something light). I would work out my legs the same day. Don't go crazy; save Tuesday and Thursday for sleeping in or for making a nice breakfast for yourself. Now that my

fingers hurt from answering your questions, I'm going to
go now

Kids Make the Fattest Moms

When to pursue a tummy tuck or liposuction

Question: I have dieted and exercised until I am blue in the face. I heard you mention before that you don't believe plastic surgery is the answer, but when diet and exercise fail to improve certain areas, especially after childbirth, and not being able to tighten your stomach back to where it was prior to childbirth or not being able to improve the saddle bags when would be the right time to pursue a tummy tuck or liposuction, as working out will not do it? Thank you!

~ *Stephanie*

Answer: I'm not necessarily sure you've worked out until you were actually blue in the face, maybe a little red, but not blue. If you were blue in the face you'd be dead and not asking me this question.

This question always comes up and I'm not a big fan of plastic or cosmetic surgery as you have pointed out. I say do everything you possibly can to build and strengthen the muscle underneath, consult with either me personally or another qualified fitness professional to see if you have done everything possible, then call a reputable plastic surgeon. There are some cases, very few mind you, that the skin stretches (where stretch marks are evident) that the skin doesn't come back and it looks like flab but is actually loose skin. Understand that I am by no means a physician and can't ever speak beyond the scope of my practice. Just do me a favor: Don't go through all of this trouble to improve your body and go on having two more kids. It's just plain annoying, to say the least.

Desperately seeking reason

Question: I had a baby 18 months ago and have had a really, really hard time losing the extra weight. I have 45 lbs. more to loose. I started Weight Watchers 4 months ago and have lost nothing. I have been to my doctor and a dietician. I work out RELIGIOUSLY 4 - 5 times a week, alternating cardio and weights. I watch what I eat and stay between 1200 - 1500 kcals per day. Please help; I am desperate.

~ Kristen

Answer: First of all getting pregnant does not give you an excuse to eat like you're going to the chair. For you ladies out there that are thinking about getting pregnant, you are not supposed to gain more than thirty-five pounds during your pregnancy. If you do it will make taking the fat off so much harder. That is what has happened to you, Kristen. I'm not sure what your workout is, because you obviously haven't told me. But if you are working out RELIGIOUSLY, then it seems to me that it could be hormonal. Sometimes it takes up to 18 months for the body to re-regulate itself and get back on track.

Most doctors won't tell you that but that's what I'm here for. I know this is going to sound absolutely nuts but I would stop working out for the next week and then start up again. I think the stress of the weight is causing some imbalance in your body. I know I'm going to get a billion e-mails over this but too bad. Take the week off and keep eating sensibly and start your workout up again. You also probably started working out again a little too early and that may have caused some energy system problems. This can be fixed by easing back into life after pregnancy.

Can't seem to get motivated after having 3 kids

Question: I know this is probably a stupid question but I'm lazy. I never had to worry about working out while growing up. I could eat anything I wanted and stayed active through color guard. I'm tired all the time and can't seem to get motivated after having 3 kids; I went from 105 lbs to 170 lbs. Can you suggest a way to motivate myself and is it possible to maybe not lose all the weight but get rid of the weight I gained especially in the stomach region?

~ Shannon

Answer: You would be absolutely correct to say this is a stupid question. If you are self-admittedly lazy, what kind of miracle could I pull out of my hat, especially in a paragraph or two that could get you off your lazy ass? I'm really not sure. I think I've said this before but it's worth repeating. Your three kids should be motivation enough to get off your ass and do something. Being around and having the capacity to watch them grow up and play sports or attend recitals would give me the motivation to begin and stick with a program. As for you being tired all the time, that comes from being inactive. The less we do, the less we want to do. Our bodies are great at adapting; if we do work the body will adapt and give us the strength and the energy to do more work. More than anything, do this for yourself and stop your whining.

My whole life I've been itty-bitty

Question: I'm 20 years old and I just had a baby 8 months ago, and I can't seem to lose the extra weight. Before I was pregnant I only weighed 102 lbs and I'm 5 feet tall, now I weigh 135 lbs. People are always asking if I'm pregnant again. My whole life I've been itty-bitty without even trying so now that I need to try I don't know how. Do you have any advice??

~ *Tiffany*

Answer: If you're still 135 lbs after eight months you must have been eating for twenty. Are you sure there isn't another kid still in there? Wow! Well, Tiffany you got the "curse of the skinny woman." You probably tortured all your friends when you were in school eating pork rinds and ice cream all day long and telling them "I can eat anything I want." Well, your friends got their revenge. Someone used a little mojo and asked the Gods to make you fat. And now you're asking me to lift that curse. Here's my advice: Stop eating as if you were going to the electric chair and begin an exercise program that stresses resistance training to help build muscle because from what it sounds like to me is that you're lean mass deficient (muscle). Five exercises I recommend in this order are:

- Lunges (long stride) same leg no less than 25 repetitions
- Jumping Jacks (as many as you can do up to 35)
- Pushups or Negative Pushups until your dead
- Jumping Jacks (as many as you can do up to 35)
- Crisscross Crunches (up to 35 repetitions)

If you're not familiar with these exercises please go to RoccoCastellano.com for the exercise demonstrations. These exercises should get you started.

They're a little saggy to say the least

Question: I am a 25-year-old mother. While I was pregnant, my breasts ballooned out to a double-D cup. Now, as I've lost most of my pregnancy weight and my breasts have gotten close to their original size, the shape is gone. They're a little saggy, to say the least. I was wondering if you could give me any pointers on how to build up my chest so the sagging is less noticeable. I'd rather not consider surgery. Thanks.

~ Lani

Answer: Saggy breasts, the most unattractive side affect of pregnancy, can be prevented. I'm glad you asked me now and not when you turned 35 after having three kids and you were able to breast-feed your baby while he/she was crawling around on the floor. Your breasts are an incredible part of your female anatomy; not only are they an important part of providing nutrients to a newborn baby, they are one of two parts that separate you from men, thank goodness.

I know this sounds a little like common sense, but an ounce of prevention is worth a pound of cure. Don't worry, I'll provide you with the pound of cure but let's first look at the prevention. Most women forget when they get pregnant that they need to support their breasts because when they grow to a size that is not natural for their bodies', gravity will always be a factor. At no time during pregnancy should they be flopping around like dolphins at SeaWorld. I know it may be uncomfortable, but buy yourself a bra that fits and allows you to breast-feed. There are no muscles within your breast; their form and structure are supported by a framework of fibrous, semi-elastic bands of tissue called

Cooper's ligaments (after the physician who first identified them). These ligaments partition the breasts into a honeycomb of interconnecting pockets, each containing mammary glands surrounded by lobules of fatty tissue. If you do not wear a supportive bra during your pregnancy, preferably with plastic supports and not under wire, gravity will allow the unnatural-size breasts to hang. As these semi-elastic (not elastic) ligaments stretch they can and usually do become like saltwater taffy. They stretch and very seldom come back to their original shape. Obviously this has happened to you and that's why you wrote me.

Here comes cure or at least a little help. Now that you've stretched your breasts beyond recognition you need to fill the bag so to speak. Most women that have this problem don't have muscle on their breastplate. The breastplate is the upper part of the chest that covers the ribs and provides cleavage. The most effective way to combat this is to add muscle to the upper chest. I recommend performing 2 sets of Flat Bench Flyes for 20 repetitions. To perform Flat Bench Flyes, lay on a bench face up, hold 3 to 5-pound dumbbells with arms straight hovering over your face, so that your hands are above your chin, lower the dumbbells laterally (sideways) until your arms become parallel to the floor, then raise your arms slowly (usually 3-4 seconds). Repeat this for 20 repetitions. And next time you get pregnant spend the extra money for a maternity bra. It's worth the money.

Fill the "Booty" bag

Question: Since my pregnancy I have lost all of my weight (I gained a lot) and pushed myself back into shape. However, I have one problem...the booty. Lunges, squats, step-ups have improved my booty considerably but it still jiggles. What else is there? I'm 36 but still think I should be able to be solid again. Help!

~ Booty

Answer: Are you related to the Funkadelic musician "Bootsy"? Maybe not, but what's a letter between friends... Booty you're killing me. You should already be solid again. 36, please! What are you doing gaining so much weight during your pregnancy? Listen ladies, and that means you too Booty, you are not supposed to gain more than 35 lbs; anymore just makes you a fat pregnant women busting out of places not intended to fit into maternity clothes. Your "booty" jiggles because you filled the bag too much and the skin grew to accommodate the amount of fat you allowed to invade your backside. If you want to keep the size of your "booty" you need to fill the bag (the skin of your butt) with muscle. If you want your "booty" smaller, then you need to exercise but be a little patient so that the body will know that it doesn't need the extra skin and will tighten on its own. But believe me it's no quick process. The exercises you're doing aren't bad but I would stop doing squats, especially after being pregnant, because squats tend to widen the hips. I can hear the e-mail inbox fill as I write this from all those women whose trainers have them doing squats -- I can't wait. I would incorporate an exercise called mountain climbers to help lift and round out the "booty" to its old bootylicious

130

state. Keep up the good work but do me a favor and get a new handle, please.

1.3 pounds fat loss safely

Question: I just gave birth to baby number 4 (ages 2 months, 14 months, 6 & 7). It is hard to find time to exercise and wanted to know what kind of exercises I can do that are fast and will give results. I just need to tone up my mid section and thighs.

~ *Julie*

Answer: Why the hell does everyone write me with questions that sound like yours? It drives me nuts. I want to ask you a question: How long did it take to get fat? You've basically been pregnant for more than two years and with that you probably have been eating for two instead of you and an embryo. Nothing is fast! If you think it is, then you're an idiot. Yes, I know, I'm being mean... boo "friggin" hoo! I'm singling you out but I want the reading public out there to also realize that if you want it fast you're the perfect candidate for the robber barons such as Gunthy-Renker. Yep, that's right, the people you see whose names appear after almost every infomercial. Stop buying this crap! It doesn't give you the results that it promises -- ever. Most programs that are based in truth can usually deliver a 1.3 lb fat loss. Remember, I said fat loss, not weight loss, per week on average. And yes, I know you heard that you can lose up to 2 lbs a week safely, but look at the statement closely, it says "up to" 2 lbs safely. It's more like 1.3 lbs and that's what most good trainers will guarantee that you will lose.

I was thinking it over and I'm not going to give you exercises that will only target the midsection and thighs because I want you to work the whole body because yours and everyone's body should work in tandem with itself. So I have decided to give everyone who signs up for a free food journal a free boot camp workout card also. Go to <u>roccocastellano.com/free-food-journal</u> and sign up for a free food journal and you'll also get the workout free. Just in time for summer. Don't say I never gave you anything.

You really don't enjoy looking like a Marsupial?

Question: Rocco, I am 5 feet 9 inches tall, slim build with a small pouch in the stomach that I held onto after I had my daughter 2 years ago. Can you recommend exercises I can do to lose the pouch and tone my body without losing weight? I weigh 140 pounds. Thanks a lot.

~ Charlotte

Question # 2: My question is this...and I am sure you have been asked dozens of times. I have 3 kids... 1 set of twins and a single. The C-sections that I had to have and the weight gain with having a multiple birth have left my stomach and abs in a very non-desirable state. Sit-ups... crunches... I have done millions. I can't retain the muscles that they cut through. I am cut from naval down, not bikini. Suggestions? Prayers? Lypo? Tummy tuck? I am desperate here. Give me some starters. I am very active. Play softball 3 days a week. Walk, play with the kids... eat decent. Help me get out of the mid-section nightmare.

Kiera

Answer: What's the matter, you two don't enjoy looking like a marsupial? It's all right, not everyone does except maybe a kangaroo, and to tell you the truth I don't even think they do.   The whole pregnancy thing drives me crazy because most women who get pregnant think their bodies are supposed to snap right back to pre-pregnancy shape. That ain't happening. The pouch problem stems from the fact that the muscles of your abdomen were stretched almost to another galaxy and decided to stay there. Most people think that sit-ups or crunches will do the trick, but it only makes the problem worse. You have stretched a muscle called the transverse abdominus, which is a muscle that helps keep your organs from spilling out of you and contracts your belly. The only way to work this muscle is to exercise it the way it's supposed to be used, by contracting it. Look in the mirror and try to only suck in the bottom portion of your belly; don't suck in the top. When you suck it in hold it for 15 seconds, let go and do it again, and repeat this process for 2 minutes. Keep practicing this and you'll be ready for that scoop-bottom swimsuit this summer.

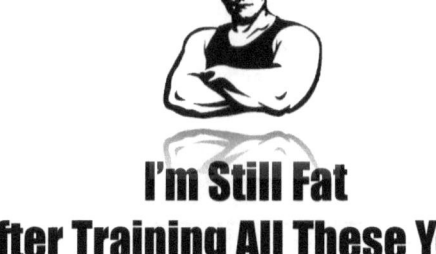

I'm Still Fat
After Training All These Years

If it doesn't learn, it will never burn...

Question: Over the last year, I have been consistently exercising and eating a healthful diet. I am 5 ft. 3in, and have gone from 175lbs. to 135lbs. My goal is 130lbs. I walk on my treadmill (4.1mph) with varying inclines 5 days per week and jog 2 miles the other 2 days. I also have a 30-minute weight-lifting routine that I do 4 days per week. I have cut back to 1200 calories - 6 small meals per day, and still can't seem to get down to my goal weight. Any advice?

~ *Katherine*

Answer: This is going to be hard for you to believe, but you won't lose anymore weight unless it's muscle. You have told me that your weight is 135 and you're only taking in 1200 calories. This will never give you the fat loss you desire since your basal metabolism is about 1350 calories, which means that just to lie in bed and not move around at all, you need to be taking in a minimum of 1350 calories per day. If you add exercise into the mix it will be significantly more. This is what the idiotic diet doctors and restrictive diets promoters want to sell you, but your body needs to learn how to burn fuel. If it doesn't learn, then it will never burn and you're stuck being fat. The small meal thing is great, but start putting more food that is nutrient dense and don't worry too much about the caloric intake unless it is pure fat and sugar. If you're taking in the proper calories you'll be capable of working out harder and getting the results you desire. If at all possible please contact a licensed dietician or nutritionist. They can really help you create a sensible eating program that can work for you.

I might as well be a fortune teller

Question: Hi Rocco!! I was just wondering if you could help me figure out what I'm doing wrong here: I work out three or four times a week where I run about 4 or 5 miles and lift weights also. I try to stay away from junk foods as much as possible yet my weight still seems to be going up. How can I change my workout so that I can LOSE weight?

~ Kate

Answer: These are the type of questions I hate. I think you have mixed me up with the gypsy fortuneteller on the boardwalk in Atlantic City. Let me see if I can shake my crystal ball and find an answer for you. Shake... Shake. I may have to put new batteries in it. For some reason it's not giving me anything. My mistake, it's not the crystal ball I need, it's the mind reading powers the witch doctors of South Africa instilled in me. Here, let me start channeling the great fitness spirit; maybe he can help me. Oooh great one! Descend upon me the powers to figure out what the hell she wants me to tell her. O.K., O.K. wow that was a trip! Well, he told me to tell you that you really need to give me more information if you want a real answer. Man that was exhausting!

Swimming is the worst exercise for fat loss.

Question: I'm extremely overweight and out of shape. To get back in shape, I have been swimming daily for cardio for about 6 months. I'm feeling better, but not getting much of a result. I'd like to get back into weight training.... how would you recommend I start off? It's been so long since I did a regular routine with weights.
~ Kylie

Answer: Swimming is the worse exercise for fat loss. When you swim breaststroke or backstroke, you're burning about the same number of calories as a fast walk or a slow jog. However, for some reason, swimming appears to be less effective than other forms of exercise at promoting weight loss.

Research published in the American Journal of Sports Medicine shows that in the absence of a controlled diet, swimming has little or no effect on fat loss.

Most swimmers notoriously have higher body fat and to combat this are given on-land exercise to help take fat off such as running or cycling. But most importantly they're given a resistance training program. In order to take fat off you need to boost your metabolism and resistance training, especially one that promotes eccentric work (letting the weight down slowly), will help to build muscle and reduce fat.

So, what does all of this have to do with swimming? Most of the work your body does in the water involves concentric muscle actions. There's virtually no eccentric work there at all. Because of this, I'm guessing that swimming has only a minor impact on your metabolic rate after exercise.

Any form of exercise, be it swimming, walking or weight training, is good if the alternative is doing nothing. A mixture of some form of resistance exercise and cardiovascular exercise is better, while combining interval exercise and resistance -- in my opinion at least -- is the best way to get in shape.

I hear the word "Core"...

Question: I'm an early 30-something male. A year ago I realized I was very out of shape and lacking any muscle tone in my core and lower body. I got a mountain bike and began riding religiously every weekend on the trail in Loveland. I am now riding 26 miles (in 2 hours time) once or twice a week and feel like I have attained a respectable level of lower body strength. My lower torso still needs help. I chose the bike because I can't stand working with stationary machines. What do you recommend for mid section/lower back strengthening exercise? Thank you so much for any consideration for an answer.

~ John

Answer: I love the way people use all these goofy fitness buzz words like... Core. Fitness enthusiasts as well as fitness professionals really need to stop making stuff up to sound cool. When I hear the word "core" I always think of an apple and it's usually the thing I'm throwing out. I'm happy to hear that you got off your ass and started to do something to get yourself into shape. You're better off than nearly three quarters of the people out there that are still fat and stupid. So kudos to you. My favorite exercise to hit your midsection (lower back and abdominals) is the crisscross crunch. To perform this exercise lie flat on your back with your knees bent and feet flat on the floor. Place your hands behind your head keeping your arms perfectly flat. While keeping your arms back bring your left elbow outside your right knee, slowly come back down and bring your right elbow to the outside of your left knee and repeat this for

20 – 30 repetitions. Pretty basic and simple, and that's the way it should be. Look ma, no buzz words!

Walking on the Treadmill seems dreadfully boring

Question: I for the life of me cannot get motivated to get back in shape.

I'm in my mid 20's and spent most of my teen years dancing and cheerleading, which kept me in a nice size 2-4, which is good for me b/c I'm not very tall. The thing is, since I no longer do those things, walking on a treadmill etc. seems dreadfully boring and tedious, so I am now a 4 pushing a 6 and I am sure it will just keep going because I don't really deprive myself of eating good food. I need a kick-start to get motivated because I am still a relatively small person, but the idea of a bathing suit makes me cringe, which is ridiculous.

Do you have any suggestions for someone that's not interested in conventional exercise, because aside from vanity I realize that it is so unhealthy for my body not to get any physical activity?

I really would like to tone up and lose around 10 pounds and I will do whatever it takes -- I just don't know what to do to maximize the results and stay interested until the results are visible. Any suggestions???

~ Casey

Answer: I have a million suggestions, but first let me tell you, stop making excuses for not having an imagination. If you don't like conventional exercise then figure out what unconventional exercise you would like. Rock climbing for instance is an awesome workout, salsa dancing and boot camp style workouts, there are so many group style activities out there, and maybe yoga can tickle your fancy. It sounds to me like you need to be in more of a social atmosphere where people are involved.

More often than not you go to the gym and everyone's got their iTunes plugged in their ears to help isolate them from the world, keeping them from having to interact. I applaud your need for interactive exercise. Go take a class, maybe take up a martial art, and kick some ass. You can have fun and exercise at the same time.

Walking 60 minutes a day not enough?

Question: Rocco, I've been walking for 60 minutes a day every morning to get in shape because I don't have enough time to go to the gym. I did fast walking more than 3 months, but my weight is unchanged yet...Do you think the walking is good to get in shape and fitness?

~ Kim

Answer: In a word no, but if I only gave one-word answers, askROCCO wouldn't be much of a column now, would it? I say no, because people like you waste an hour every morning not hitting fitness goals. You have just admitted to me that you walk an hour every morning because you don't have time to go to the gym, ohhh... but you have time to walk for an hour. I don't know, maybe the locker room stench is getting to me but I think I have stated in the past that an hour is more than enough time to work out. If you have an hour of time 6 days a week try this: 30 minutes of resistance training: Jumping Jacks, Pushups, Lunges, Crunches, Mountain Climbers.

Do these in a circuit style, one set jumping jacks, then pushups, lunges, etc. then start over with the Jumping Jacks and repeat this three times. It's a hell of a good time. When you're finished with the circuit then go for your walk, but while you're walking, try a little jog until you get tired and then walk again, and if you feel up to it jog again. Keep doing that until the half hour's up, go home, shower and get your ass to work. Do this three times a week and I just saved you three hours a week to do something else besides wandering around aimlessly like fourth-class mail.

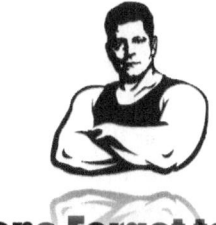

Someone Forgot to Tell You
Fitness is Free

Working out the same time every day?

Question: Does it matter if I don't work out at the same time every day? During the week it's more convenient for me to work out after work around 5pm; however on the weekends I work out in the mornings around 9am. Will switching times hurt my workout?

~ Jenn

Answer: Actually I'm not sure how to answer that question because it sounds like you're working out an awful lot, but I won't bitch at you too bad. At least you're working out. I have heard and read differing views on this subject and I won't go into them here. My opinion is that if you feel comfortable working out at a certain time and you feel you're getting a good workout then it's fine.

Many people enjoy working out in the morning before work, some in the afternoon and others at night. Whatever allows you to get the best workout is what you do. I hate the trainers or people that preach that you have to work out at specific times to get the best results. Find a time, get it done and go on with the rest of your life.

Don't tell my clients or I'll be eating cat food

Question: I'm a very poor. Poor with a capital **P**. So, a membership to the gym is out. I'm also a mom to a very adventurous crawler that lives to eat the cat's food while I'm not looking. My fitness solution is to walk for about an hour daily carrying my 20-pound cat food-craving child. I am working on becoming fit, and need to lose about 30 pounds. Along with a healthy diet, will this work?

~ SJ

Answer: I'm glad you wrote me, because no one should actually have to pay for fitness and well-being (don't tell my clients that or I'll be eating cat food). To answer your question: NO. Your current program is lacking several real fitness components. First I'd like you to pick the cat food dish up off the floor and put it where Spider baby can't get at it. Then put down Spider baby, preferably in a crib or playpen with a dome roof and a bunch of toys to keep him occupied for only five minutes. In order for you to lose fat you need to gain muscle first, so let's perform some muscle-building exercises, and then when you walk you'll just be burning fat. Do these exercises before you take your walk.

- 50 jumping jacks with your arms perfectly straight (if you don't know how to do a Jumping Jack, go to askrocco.com to download workouts with exercise illustrations).
- 25 Lunges each leg (do not alternate, that is for wusses).
- Stairs, two steps at a time and come down that flight walking one step at a time (do not run: that would be stupid, you may fall and want to blame

me, so again don't). Do eight flights of about 16
– 18 steps (8 – 9 double steps).

- If you can do push-ups, do 20; if not perform 15
negative push-ups (if you don't know how look
in the back of this book).
- 50 more jumping jacks and go for your walk.
Without the kid on your hip, we don't want you
looking like Quasimoto. Good Luck.

So many books, videos, magazines... it's a bit overwhelming!

Question: What's the best thing an overweight couch potato can do to start being more physically active and lose weight? There are so many books, videos, magazines, websites, infomercials, and it is all a bit overwhelming sometimes. I get the cardio thing, I think - walking, biking, running, things to get the heart beating fast. But what about strength training? Is joining a gym the only way to get stronger? Thanks!!

~ *Ann*

Answer: The first thing I would do is throw away your couch and your television. This would keep you from coming home from work and plopping down on the couch, turning on the tube and eating the shit you have in your fridge. Sometimes I recommend people just take their television and move it to another room like the bedroom, so that you only watch it at night when you go to sleep. If the couch is your problem than you really need to get off of your ass. The most important thing to understand is that going from couch potato to non-couch potato is a lifestyle change. Lifestyle changes require adjustments in your attitude. I don't care if I give you a million books, tapes, etc., you still won't be motivated until you look inside and find that something that drives you. Now getting to the strength training question, no, joining a gym is not the only way to get stronger. I would recommend consulting a fitness professional before starting anything since you've been inactive so long. If you go into my archives at cincinnati.com you'll find past columns on my five favorite exercises. They can be done at home, outside, the office or even church if you're so inclined.

Education is the key to motivation

Question: Just wondering… have YOU ever struggled with your weight?
Have you always been fit all of your life?

How did you get started… and stick with… a routine of weight loss, working out and eating right… and how the HECK do you always stay so motivated?
~ *JC*

Answer: To tell you the truth, I never had a great weight problem but when I was young I had to shop in the "husky" section of the clothes stores and in my 20's I bulked up to 240 lbs. Keeping motivated is a very tricky thing because it all depends on what your motivation is for wanting to lose the fat in the first place. Everything has got to come from within. You cannot try to do this for any reason but to be a better you. Your attitude needs to change from being reactive to being proactive. An example of this would be: "That girl won't date me because she thinks I'm too fat, I need to lose weight" to "I think my weight has created insecurity within me I want to make a change." If you know how to ask the right questions you'll get better answers. If you look in the mirror and ask yourself "Why am I so fat?" your brain will tell you "because you eat like a fat pig and you're a lazy slob." I don't think that's the type of answer you would want to hear, but it happens all the time. A more appropriate question would be, "What do I have to do to make myself less fat?" Don't worry, your brain may fumble around for a moment but it will find the answer and it usually goes something like this; "I need to educate myself a little more about this exercise and eating thing." Once you have established that you need help and get a proper education (e.g. Fitness Seminars, Qualified Fitness Professional, and Licensed Nutritionists) it's much easier to keep motivated.

The problem most of us have is that no one actually knows how bad we are to our bodies and how out of balance they are. When you start feeling, looking and thinking better, motivation isn't necessarily a problem anymore, the problem becomes finding more challenging things to do. Education is the key to motivation, so start asking the right questions and see how your life will change for the better.

Even if you drank the Kool Aid, it's not too late.

Question: Hello, I'm 5ft 9in and weigh 120lbs I do not want to lose weight only tone what I have. I recently had a baby and want to get rid of the extra skin. I bought an Easy Shaper and have been using it now for 1 month with little or no results. I am not on a diet because I don't want to lose weight; I follow the video, and do same exercises. I'm not sure if the equipment is not targeting the areas I'm trying to work on enough, which would be abs and legs, or if I really should be watching what I eat. I have never counted the calorie intake due to never having a weight problem, but now I'm unsure if I need to get better results from the workouts. Please help.
~ Tonia, Adams County

Answer: Tonia, you drank the Kool Aid and I'm sorry. Some of you will get the reference and some of you won't. Those of you who don't will drink the same Kool Aid. You actually believed this statement and paid with your credit card in 3 easy payments:

"Easy Shaper was designed by a woman for women, the Easy Shaper targets the seven areas woman want to work the most. Easy Shaper tones your arms and back. Easy Shaper sculpts your hips, buns and thighs. Easy Shaper tightens your abdominals and obliques – All on one simple machine that is small enough to store just about anywhere."

(Taken from the actual Easy Shaper advertisement)

Sweetheart, of course you're not getting results BECAUSE YOU'RE NOT ACTUALLY SUPPOSED TO GET RESULTS. You're just supposed to buy the stupid thing and put it in your basement with the rest of the garbage you will eventually set out for the trash or a garage sale. Let me ask you a question: Do you think anything that costs $165.00 with all those promises will actually give you results? No, no, let me answer it for you, no, really let me help you. OF COURSE NOT! And do you know why? I'll answer this one for you also: because it costs less then $40 dollars to make in Tiawan. You're basically paying $165.00 for a Thighmaster, and you know how much those things worked. Suzanne Sommers is still laughing all the way to the bank on that joke. I'm going to let you and everyone else out there that has bought something as stupid as the Easy Shaper in on a little secret: Fitness is Free! It doesn't cost anything to perform lunges, does it? It doesn't cost anything to perform mountain climbers or walk steps or I don't know: a crunch, sit-up and a host of other exercises that don't require your credit card number and shipping charges.

My gym doesn't have a chin up bar

Question: In addition to wanting to lose weight, be healthy and feel good, I have a weird fitness goal: I'd like to be able to do chin-ups like Linda Hamilton did in *Terminator II*. When I was little, I couldn't do a single chin-up in gym class--I just hung onto the bar. Now that I'm a 25-year-old woman, I'd like to try and do this. My gym doesn't have a chin-up bar so I guess I'll go to the park down the street, but what other exercises do you recommend to get my upper body strong enough to accomplish my goal?

~ *Alecia*

Answer: Alecia! I love these types of questions. I do have to ask you though, what makes you think if you couldn't do a chin-up when you were a little munchkin you can even think about doing one now? I do like your determination and if you're up for the challenge I'll help you out. First, tell those cheap bastards at your gym to buy a chin up bar or go buy one yourself. I think they sell them at any fitness store for twenty bucks or something close to that. Now that you've got something to grab on to I want you to place a chair underneath the bar you've just acquired. Stand on the chair and grab the bar with both hands shoulder width apart. Hopefully your chin is above the bar at this point in time. Bend your knees so your feet don't touch the chair anymore. Lower yourself slow enough to count to six until your arms are straight. Place your feet back on the chair, stand up and repeat lowering yourself as many times as you can without your arms ripping themselves out of the socket. This is called a negative chin up. If you keep practicing this exercise you will eventually develop enough strength to pull yourself up. Good luck and don't forget to write. Hopefully, you'll be back! (Sorry I can't do the Arnold accent on paper.)

I can't afford to go to the gym...

Question: I have lost 60 lbs and don't know where to begin and what exercises I can use to tone up all around, example hips, stomach, arms. I can't afford to go to the gym to exercise and would like to do it at home.
~ Dorothy

Answer: I hate these questions because everyone is going to want to know how you lost the 60 pounds without exercise. Now since you probably feel like an empty sack of potatoes and have excess skin hanging on you like you're melting you want me to give you exercises after the fact. Like playing Monday morning quarterback, oops I think I forgot something. First, you should have consulted me or another fitness professional before losing all that weight. Second, there are five exercises that I always recommend to anyone that wants to start an exercise program when they can't afford to go to the gym. For those out there that didn't know, fitness is free you don't need to spend money to get into shape.
1) Jumping Jacks 25-50 reps
2) Push-ups or negative push-ups (as many as you can)
3) Stairs (two at a time) or Lunges
4) Mountain Climbers (run in place on all fours)
5) Crunches with your feet on a chair.

Because your joints are probably a little beat up from not doing any strength training before losing the weight I would not recommend walking until you have strengthened your lower body joints (i.e. hips, knees, ankles). The exercises provided will help to develop symmetry and strengthen auxiliary muscles. Next time gain the muscle then lose the fat.

Is there a reason you're planning for rough times?

Question: I am interested in beginning a workout plan. I am getting older and I realize that now is a better time than ever to get in shape for the rough times ahead. Would you be able to recommend a good workout routine for me? I don't want to walk into the gym and be dumbfounded about what to do there. I am 5'2", about 110lbs. I want to focus on a full-body workout.

~ *Tasha*

Answer: Is there a reason you are planning for rough times? Are you anticipating going into battle, maybe the battle of the bulge? You may have to kick someone's ass in the near future. I don't know but it sounds intriguing. There are many workouts that could be done outside the gym that would constitute a full-body workout. But because you asked I'll give you one. You wouldn't be the first person to walk into a gym dumbfounded, walk around confused and then walk back out, never to return because people who own the gyms forgot long ago about customer service. Getting back to the full-body workout, for the gym I recommend:

- Hip adduction & abduction for 25 reps* (it's the exercise machine that spreads your legs out)
- Leg Press (not the hip sled, the horizontal press) for 25 reps
- Seated hamstring curl 20 reps (sit on the machine and pull your lower legs towards your butt)
- Incline dumbbell chest press (lie on incline at 45-degree angle and press upward over your

nose so that the dumbbells are directly over your nose) for 15-20 reps
- Lat pull-downs (the machine with a wide bar connected to a cable, grab the bar with palms facing down, lean back a little, so you don't smash your face with the bar, pull the bar down to the top of your chest) for 15-20 reps
- Dumbbell lateral raises (grab the dumbbells at your side and raise them sideways to just over the tops of your ears and then back down) for 20 reps

Finish it all off with some cross crunches with your legs raised (make sure you curl, bringing your rib cage to your pelvis) until you can't do anymore. So here it is. You didn't give me enough information, that's why there are no weights included. It may take a little trial and error before you get the correct weight for an intense enough workout. With that said get your ass to the gym.

* Repetitions

Should I consult a Personal Trainer?

Question: I have worked really hard to lose over 70 pounds last year. I keep trying to find a maintenance program that works. Everything, I try... I start putting the weight back on.

I don't want to continue working out 1 hour 6 days a week. I would love to cut it down to 3 or 4 days and maybe only 40 minutes. My diet is the same as when I was losing weight.

Should I consult a personal trainer? I really don't have the cash to do that but I am getting burned out on exercise. Do I need to cut my food down even further?
~ *Betty*

Answer: Well... Betty, here's the problem. You're not doing one of two things consistently, either eating sensibly or exercising. If you're doing both of them simultaneously it's very hard to gain the weight back. So to answer part of your question, if you're not eating sensibly then you will have to continue working out 6 days a week for 1 hour. Do not cut your food intake down (unless you're eating for a family of four); just make better choices in the food you take in i.e. more vegetables and fruit.

Sometimes after losing so much weight the body will gain a little back because it's trying to re-regulate. This shouldn't be too much of a problem, but most people get scared to death. If you gain 5 pounds back it's all right. You can't keep losing weight without plateauing at least once; the body doesn't work like that.

If you're getting burned out on exercise I would try some other form of physical activity that you may find less boring. The problem is most of us need to get at least forty-five minutes of vigorous exercise a day to stay healthy. You can cut down the time of exercise if you increase the intensity when it pertains to strength training. If you're not doing a strength-training program you need to do one and that I would consult a personal trainer on, but make sure they have dealt with people with your problem and not some pretty boy or girl that looks good in shorts.

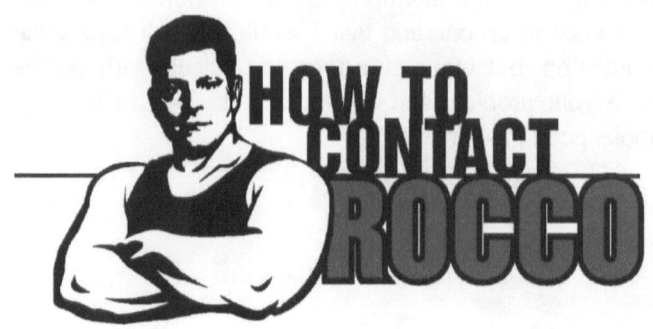

A selection of products and services intended to help individuals face the facts about there fatness are available. Look over the current list on the following page and contact askROCCO Media for more information or to place an order.

askROCCO Media welcomes your feedback. Please feel free to share your story of fat loss and your experience by emailing or writing us.

Visit askROCCO on the World Wide Web

If you are interested in learning more and you have access to the Internet come visit us at:

RoccoCastellano.com

You'll find complete information on all the products and services we offer and you'll have access to the latest updates on the topic of FAT.

---

iTunes Audios

These audios speak directly to your circumstances. They can be listened to in the privacy of your home, car or while exercising. They cover some of he most poignant issues you might be facing. *Narrated by Rocco Castellano*

Seminars/Workshops askROCCO Live Events

Seminars, workshops and askROCCO Live events led by Rocco Castellano are coming to your town, company or school.

Fitness Professionals

If you're looking for new concepts to help you make more money, help your clients get better results or you want to participate in one of my *askROCCO* **LIVE** events for personal trainers I would like to include you in my network of trainers. Only currently certified personal trainers need respond.

On The Internet:

Contact me by e-mail:
rocco@roccocastellano.com

By Mail:

askROCCO Media, LLC
8022 South Rainbow Blvd
Suite 219
Las Vegas, NV 89139

For information on askROCCO Media seminars and
consulting services, call or email me
Monday through Saturday,
12 pm to 7pm. PST
702.708.2847 or
1.212.729.6531
rocco@roccocastellano.com